T0210945

HEALTH,
POLITICS,
AND
REVOLUTION
IN CUBA
SINCE 1898

HEALTH, POLITICS, AND REVOLUTION IN CUBA SINCE 1898

KATHERINE HIRSCHFELD

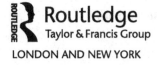

Routledge
Taylor & Francis Group

LONDON AND NEW YORK

First published 2009 by Transaction Publishers

Published 2017 by Routledge
2 Park Square, Milton Park, Abingdon, Oxon OX14 4RN
711 Third Avenue, New York, NY 10017, USA

Routledge is an imprint of the Taylor & Francis Group, an informa business

Library of Congress Catalog Number: 2006040263

Library of Congress Cataloging-in-Publication Data

Hirschfeld, Katherine.
  Health, politics, and revolution in Cuba : 1898-2005 / Katherine Hirschfeld.
      p. cm.
   Includes bibliographical references and index.
   ISBN 0-7658-0344-5 (alk. paper)
   1. Medical policy—Cuba—History—20th century. 2. Medical care—
Political aspects—Cuba—History—20th century. 3. Public health—Political
aspects—Cuba—History—20th century. I. Title.

RA395.C9H57 2006
362.1097291—dc22   2006040263

ISBN 13: 978-1-4128-0863-7 (pbk)

Contents

Acknowledgments

This book has been almost ten years in the making, and would never have reached completion if not for tremendous help from a number of people. In Atlanta, Peter Brown, Claire Sterk, and Peggy Barlett were all exceptionally kind and generous with their time in reading early versions of my dissertation, as well as helping me stay focused on writing through a very difficult post-fieldwork meltdown. Juan Del Aguila and Melvin Konner also read early chapters and offered advice and encouragement at crucial junctures. Charles Rutheiser has made vital intellectual and personal contributions from the very earliest days of the project. The administrative staff of Emory University's anthropology department (Amy-Lynn Caplan, Dee Shriver, and Shirley Sabo) were also outstanding in managing the complexities of research grants and fieldwork in an embargoed country. The dissertation fieldwork was funded by a small grant from the Massey Foundation in Atlanta, as well as a doctoral dissertation grant from the Wenner-Gren Foundation.

During my early write-up period, the social science students and faculty at Agnes Scott College (particularly Martha Rees, Brenda Hoke, and Yvonne Newsome) provided me with a warm and supportive work environment that revitalized a good deal of my passion for anthropology. Although they would probably disclaim any contribution to my intellectual life, Tommy Futch and the other folks of Laughing Matters improvisational comedy troupe contributed much by restoring my sense of humor during the dissertation years, as did my Atlanta housemates Eric Litwin and Kevin Caran. Recently that role has been taken over by my husband, Corson Hirschfeld, whose creativity and humor inspire me on a daily basis.

For the archival phase of this project, I am also deeply grateful to all of the archivists at National Archives in College Park, Maryland and Washington, DC who have helped me track down odd minutiae of Cuban history. Marty McGann has been a particularly outstanding resource for archival material.

At the University of Oklahoma I have been blessed with the best of all possible worlds: supportive friends and colleagues in the department of anthropology, and generous research funding in the College of Arts and Sciences. For their help in negotiating all of these things, I am grateful to Drs. Patricia Gilman, Morris Foster, and Lesley Rankin-Hill, as well as Kim Tiger and Wanda Downs for administrative support. Peter Cahn merits special thanks for his insightful comments on one early section of this work, for dancing at my wedding, and for timely infusions of moral support.

Many others people have helped this project along, including Paul Hollander, who graciously read a very early draft of the manuscript. Howard Stein has been an ongoing source of inspiration, as well as a delightful friend and mentor. And I owe a long-standing debt of gratitude to Irving Louis Horowitz, whose generosity and encyclopedic knowledge of Cuba have saved me from grievous errors on more than one occasion. (Any remaining errors, of course, are fully my own.)

Unfortunately, the people to whom I owe the most must unfortunately remain unacknowledged. These are the Cubans themselves, who took tremendous risks to speak openly with me, and who always responded to my painfully naive questions with graciousness, warmth and humor. It is to them that this book is dedicated.

Introduction

Cuba and Medical Anthropology

In academia, one hears only good things about the Cuban health care system. Medical historians, anthropologists, physicians and public health researchers have all written favorable assessments of the Castro regime's health initiatives for many years. The 1959 revolution and transition to socialism have been credited with rapidly transforming Cuba's mortality profile (Danielson, 1977; Danielson, 1979; Danielson, 1981; Elling, 1989; Gilpin, 1991; Waitzkin, 1983), eliminating class-based disparities in health status and access to health care (Chomsky, 2000; Feinsilver, 1993; Nayeri, 1995; Singer and Baer, 1995; Whiteford and Martinez, 2000; Spiegel and Yassi, 2004) and "revolutionizing" medical practice and medical science in a number of positive ways (Baer, Singer and Johnson, 1986; Dresang et al., 2005; Feinsilver, 1993; de Brun and Elling, 1987; Guttmacher and Danielson 1979; Santana, 1988; Swanson et al., 1995; Waitzkin and Britt, 1989; Waitzkin et al., 1997; Warman, 2001). In fact, some scholars continue to argue that despite the debilitating economic crisis brought on by the collapse of the Soviet Union, Cuba's health system remains superior to neighboring countries such as the Dominican Republic (Acosta, 1997; Chomsky, 2000; Herrera-Valdés, 2005; Waitzkin et al., 1997; Whiteford, 2000; Whiteford and Martinez, 2001).

Most of these works use statistics to highlight Cuba's health achievements. Before the Revolution, infectious diseases were common, infant mortality was high and life expectancy was low. Shortly after the Castro regime took power, these negative trends were reversed—infectious diseases are now controlled, infant mortality is extremely low and life expectancy is on a par with countries such as Sweden and

1

Great Britain (Nayeri, 1995; Santana, 1988; Spiegel and Yassi, 2004; Swanson, Swanson, Gill and Walter, 1995; Waitzkin and Britt, 1989). Neighboring countries such as Puerto Rico and the Dominican Republic, on the other hand, still suffer from high infant mortality rates and outbreaks of preventable infectious diseases. If health statistics are any indication (and often they are the only indication), Cuba's approach to health care appears far superior to that of other Latin American countries.

So how did Cuba's remarkable transformation in health and disease take place? What exactly did the revolutionaries do to improve health conditions so dramatically? According to most scholars, Cuba's socialist approach to medicine has transformed the interface between the health system and the social world—integrating doctors into the community, and integrating the community into medical practice. This transformation was ostensibly responsible for Cuba's health achievements: controlling or eradicating infectious diseases, and transforming Cuba's mortality profile from "underdeveloped" (high mortality from infectious disease/high infant mortality) to "developed" (mortality from chronic diseases such as heart disease or cancer). The egalitarianism of the socialist economy is also credited with reducing poverty and eliminating health disparities on the island (see Baer, 1989; Chomsky, 2000; Danielson, 1979; DeBrun and Elling, 1987; Elling, 1989; Feinsilver, 1993; Gilpin, 1991; Nayeri, 1995; Waitzkin, 1983).

Fieldwork

In 1996 I traveled to Havana for a year of dissertation field research to look at this transformation of health and medicine up close. My goal was to use anthropological research methods—long-term residence, participant observation, case studies, ethnographic interviews— to study the socialization of health and medicine in Cuba. There would be three parts to the project. First would be living and participating in everyday life in a local community for a year, with the goal of learning more about Cuban culture, and to observe the ways people behaved with respect to health and disease in their everyday lives, outside of the formal health sector. The second phase of the project would consist of formal clinic observations in at least two family doctor clinics. I would shadow these physicians during the course of their workdays so that I could get a better sense of what family medicine was like in practice. I would also conduct formal and informal interviews with family doctors, soliciting their personal reflections on Cuba's unique social medicine programs. And finally, from the local community and the clinics I would draw a series of case studies that best exemplified the social and cultural dynamics of Cuban health care. As originally conceptualized, the project was intended to document (and highlight) Cuba's achievements in social medicine.

During my time in Cuba, my opinion of the Cuban health care system underwent a dramatic transformation. The idealistic, egalitarian system I had read about in the scholarly literature seemed to bear little resemblance to the conditions I observed in my study communities. While many of the individual doctors I worked with were dedicated and caring professionals, they were forced to work within a system that was deeply politicized, authoritarian and repressive. Manipulation of health statistics for political purposes was also apparent.

A key experience in bringing about this change of perspective was my participation in the 1997 epidemic of dengue fever in Oriente Province. According to several recent publications (Kouri et al., 1998; Mendoza and Fuentes, 2001), dengue first broke out in Santiago early in January, 1997, shortly after my arrival. None of the physicians or public health personnel I was working with in Santiago, however, acknowledged the outbreak, and instead everyone repeatedly assured me that Cuba had successfully eradicated dengue. Articles in *Granma* (the official daily newspaper) claimed that "not one case" had been seen on the island since the early 1980s.

By mid-summer, the outbreak in Santiago surged into a massive epidemic—a fact I discovered only when I became sick myself and was taken (against my will) to a crowded hospital ward. Once admitted as a patient, I discovered there had been thousands of cases of dengue and hemorrhagic dengue in Santiago and its surrounding towns since early spring. This surprise was eclipsed only by the extremely poor care I received in the hospital. No physician spoke to me about my condition, mosquitoes swarmed throughout the wards, and (other than a single vitamin tablet) I was given no medications to alleviate my suffering. Nursing care was scarce, and ambulatory patients (such as myself) took care of those too sick to move. Since the epidemic was considered a state secret, an armed soldier guarded the entry to the ward. I was not allowed to telephone anyone in the United States about my condition.

After my release from the hospital, I learned that physicians in Santiago had been prohibited by law from diagnosing dengue in their patients for the duration of the epidemic. I (and everyone else with me in the dengue wards) had instead been given a diagnosis of "virosis," or a virus. Only after a dissident doctor broke the story to the international media did the Cuban government reluctantly acknowledge that there had been a dengue fever outbreak in Santiago. Both *Science* and *The Lancet* featured brief news stories, and a series of dispatches from Reuters were published on the internet through *CubaNet News* (a website that featured news reports from unofficial sources inside Cuba).

The first Reuters story appeared on June 17, a full two weeks before any notice of the epidemic in Cuba. In this article, the Cuban government acknowledged that there had been a dengue outbreak, but claimed there had only been about 750 cases detected. At this time I estimated there were at least 10,000 cases in Santiago, based on the occupancy rate of my hospital. A week after this initial report a dissident Cuban physician, Dr. Desi Mendoza, defied the government news blackout and gave a critical interview to *Diario de las Americas*. In this interview, he accused the Cuban government of showing "contempt for the lives of its citizens" in keeping the epidemic a secret. Shortly after this interview, Dr. Mendoza was arrested and charged with "disseminating counterrevolutionary propaganda" (Associated Press, November 20, 1997).

Immediately following publication of Dr. Mendoza's criticisms, the official Cuban media published its first reports of the dengue epidemic in *Sierra Maestra*. Still, no figures on the number of cases or the number of deaths were published. Subsequent news reports in the international and official Cuban media contradict one other greatly in their respective assessments of the epidemic. Shortly after Dr. Mendoza's arrest, *Granma* declared the epidemic to be "frankly eradicated" (July 11, 1997). On the same day, *Science* magazine published a story claiming there may have been as many as 30,000 cases of dengue in Santiago. According to the Washington, DC office of the Pan American Health Organization, after the epidemic the Cuban government officially reported that there had been 2,946 cases of dengue in Santiago, with 205 cases of dengue hemorrhagic fever and twelve deaths (Dr. Francisco de Paul Pinherio, personal communication). By my estimates, these official figures underestimate the true extent of the epidemic by about a factor of ten.[1]

This experience left me skeptical of official Cuban government communiqués regarding health. If the dengue epidemic was any indication, government publications were used largely to erase or obscure negative health trends on the island. The lack of competing non-governmental news outlets meant that this strategy could be quite successful—many people I met in Havana (including health officials) had no idea there had been an epidemic in Santiago. This realization led to something of a dilemma with respect to my research project, since nearly all of the anthropological literature on Cuba was based on uncritical acceptance of Cuban government health publications. If official sources were inaccurate or suspect, then so were all (or at least many) of the assumptions medical anthropologists and public health personnel had made about the health impact of the 1959 revolution. How could I use anthropological methods to explore Cuba's achievements in health and social medicine when I was no longer certain those achievements were legitimate?

There was no way I could undertake a new ethnographic research project investigating the veracity of official government sources describing health conditions on the island. Public dissent from the party line remains a serious crime in Cuba, and foreign researchers are closely watched—especially if they begin to ask the wrong kinds of questions (see Lewis, 1977; Rosendahl, 1997). In fact, soon after my release from the hospital, I was subject to several uncomfortable visits from Cuban State Security officers who questioned me about my political beliefs, my research agenda and what I intended to publish about Cuba once I returned to the United States. These encounters coincided with a new wave of repression on the island, and a series of restrictive measures were passed by the Cuban government designed to further impede informal social interactions between Cubans and foreigners. By late summer, circumstances had deteriorated to the point where I was forced to abandon my ethnographic research on the island altogether.

At that point, I did not have enough data to write a complete thesis, nor would I be able to return to Cuba to do additional fieldwork, due to my newfound skepticism about the reliability of Cuban government sources. Whatever additional research I undertook would have to be done in the United States. One option would be to continue ethnographic work with recent Cuban exiles and immigrants to assess their experiences with the socialist health system. Another would be to do historical research to critically reevaluate health conditions in Cuba prior to 1959, to better estimate the actual health impact of the 1959 revolution.

While the thought of working with exiles was appealing, I also feared the intense politicization of certain sectors of the exile leadership. At least one branch of the exile movement remains violently opposed to any contact or travel between the United States and Cuba. I had also seen several noted anthropologists make dismissive or disparaging comments about Cuban exiles and feared these prejudices might lead mainstream academics to dismiss any ethnographic research done among this population—particularly research intended to critique the health claims of the Castro government.

Revisiting History

Historical research seemed like a wiser choice. During my time in Santiago, I conducted some preliminary research in local historical archives that suggested the conventional historical narrative of health patterns in twentieth century Cuba (upon which much medical anthropology scholarship is based) is incorrect, or at least incomplete. Medical anthropologists, for instance, typically describe the time period from 1902 to 1959 as a single "pre-revolutionary" era characterized by undifferentiated suffering and disease. High rates of infant mortality and infectious disease during this time are interpreted as resulting from U.S. imperialism and the socioeconomic inequalities of capitalism. The end of imperialism and the 1959 revolution are then described as bringing about an immediate improvement in health conditions (see Waitzkin, 1983; Waitzkin and Britt, 1989; Singer and Baer, 1989; Nayeri, 1995; Simons, 1996).

Historical documents in the Santiago archives, however, implied a different series of events, a different set of political-economic forces acting to shape health conditions prior to 1959, and a more modest improvement in health conditions following the 1959 revolution. In the early twentieth century, local sanitation officials in Oriente Province frequently wrote U.S. leaders to lobby for more (not less) United States intervention in Cuba as a means to improve (not destroy) health conditions. These local professionals spoke highly of the health effects of the U.S. military occupation of Cuba following the Spanish-Cuban-American War, and negatively about national public health and sanitation programs within the Cuban government during the early republican period. They also complained about the politicization of health in the national government, and described how bitter factionalism and violence in local politics interfered with their duties and led to resurgent outbreaks of infectious disease. While the United States *economic* presence in Cuba (as represented by private corporations such as the United Fruit Company) was occasionally the subject of criticism, the United States *political* presence in Cuba (as manifest in government or military intervention under the Platt Amendment) was frequently solicited as a means to control the political violence and instability that threatened the functioning of the government health sector.

Intrigued by the discrepancies between these documents and conventional anthropological representations of Cuba's health history, I continued to do research in a number of archival collections in the United States and Havana.[2] The close historic ties that prevailed between the two countries prior to 1959 meant that health conditions were often the subject of diplomatic correspondence and journalistic reports. The United States Public Health Service also maintained a research station in Havana from the late 1800s until the abrogation of the Platt Amendment in 1933, and these officials sent monthly reports to Washington, DC detailing health and social conditions on the island. Within Cuban archives, I was able to explore papers from the Cuban Academy of Sciences, as well as internal correspondence between local sanitation chiefs and their superiors in Havana.

A New Model

This research led to the construction of an alternative health history for twentieth century Cuba that diverges from existing scholarship in medical anthropology in two major ways. The first divergence is the reconfiguration of Cuba's health history into a more accurate temporal framework, consisting of four distinct eras. Instead of a single "pre-revolutionary" period, I will argue that the time period between 1898 and 1959 should be divided as follows: 1) the later years of the War of Independence against Spain (1890s–1902); 2) the U.S. military occupations of the Island (1898–1902, and 1906–1909); 3) the Platt era (1909–1933); and 4) the Auténtico-Batista decades (1933–1959). The second area of divergence involves a critical reappraisal of the social, political and economic factors involved in configuring health trends on the island during these periods.

In other words, this work seeks to challenge several key assumptions of the medical anthropology and public health literature on Cuba. These assumptions are as follows: 1) that the term "pre-revolutionary" is meaningful as far as describing health trends between 1902 and 1959; 2) that poor health conditions prior to 1959 were due primarily to United States intervention and imperialism; and 3) that the 1959 Castro revolution represented a radical departure from earlier patterns in Cuban history, and led to an immediate, dramatic improvement in health conditions for the majority of the Cuban population.

Exploring these issues necessitates discussion of both historical and ethnographic material at multiple levels of analysis. My ethnographic fieldwork, for instance, was crucial in shifting my research focus and prompting me to take a more a critical look at the Castro regime's health claims, and to explore Cuba's health history as represented in original documents. As such, the fieldwork experience merits detailed exposition. A description of my time in Cuba is also significant in that it conveys important aspects of everyday life on the island that have often gone missing from anthropological accounts. Few anthropologists or sociologists have been allowed to conduct long-term research in Cuba, and as a result, academic writing in this area has often consisted of statistical data rather than direct experience in individual communities. While a more empirically distanced approach does offer some methodological advantages, it can also lead to a distorted analytical gaze. As Carlos Alberto Montaner has stated, "No one is capable of deducing the intimate nature of the [Cuban] revolution, the daily life it generates, from a reading of the patient and meritorious compilation of information. The ineluctable human dimension, the drama, is left out" (1981:3). To counter the mandatory ethnographic distance imposed by Cold War hostilities in the 1970s and 1980s, the first section of this work (chapters 1 through 5) is correspondingly taken up with a personal narrative of my experiences as a researcher in Cuba in the late 1990s, including my participation in the 1997 epidemic of dengue fever.

The cumulative effect of this subjective experience was to make me critically reevaluate my original assumptions about Cuba, the 1959 Revolution, and health. Before my fieldwork, I had sympathized with scholars who portrayed "revolutionary" regimes (and their health systems) as more egalitarian, more rational and more peaceful than their "imperialist" enemies. After living in Cuba, however, it was increasingly apparent that the revolutionary government in Havana was just as guilty of ideological extremism, coercion and aggression as the militant exile factions in Miami.

The dictatorial, authoritarian features of the Castro regime can be difficult to see from abroad, and the humanitarian rhetoric of the revolutionary leadership continues to inspire loyalty and support from a number of leading North American academics. But in my experience, the reality of life on the island rarely conforms to the ideals professed by Cuba's political leaders. In fact, the discrepancy between reality and ideal was often so painful and ironic that it led me to reject most of the literature that originally framed my research project.[3] This phenomenon (the rejection of Marxist theory following time spent in a Marxist regime) has been a common experience for many scholars (see Berger, 1977a; 1986; Hollander, 1983; 1998; Horowitz, 1993; Radosh, 2001), but has had little impact on the popularity of Marxism within academia. As Irving Horowitz has stated, "In eastern Europe discussions of Marxism and socialism are relegated to the world of black humor; but in the United States, with notable exceptions, the sacred texts of yesteryear are pored over with a sobriety and affectation that would well inspire religious zealots" (1993:32).

Some readers will no doubt criticize the influence of my subjective experience as a researcher in Cuba in shaping my subsequent research agenda. Is it inappropriate to let personal experiences motivate one's intellectual pursuits? Research undertaken under such circumstances is not necessarily "objective." On the other hand, recent trends in postmodern ethnography may lead others to applaud an honest discussion of the ways subjectivity and emotion shape scholarly inquiry. Did getting sick and spending time in a Cuban hospital enhance or distort my perceptions of Cuba and the Cuban health care system? Was my experience as a researcher in Cuba typical or exceptional? In my own case, I would simply note that the uniquely personal nature of anthropological fieldwork means there will never be a satisfying boundary between objective and subjective research, and these questions will always provoke debate within the profession.

The fieldwork narrative serves as an extended introduction to the revisionist health history presented in the remainder of the book. Chapter 6 begins with a discussion of health conditions during the War of

Independence against Spain in the late 1800s, in order to establish baseline health data from which to measure the subsequent progress in disease eradication through the twentieth century. Chapter 7 details the dramatic turnaround in disease rates that followed the Spanish-Cuban-American War. In the later years of the War, Cuba easily had one of the worst mortality profiles in the hemisphere. By 1909, however, this trend had become completely reversed—many infectious diseases were controlled, and mortality rates dropped dramatically. This remarkable transition occurred over the course of just a few years, and had a lasting impact on mortality in Cuba for many decades. Levels of infectious disease rose slightly during the republican period, but never again returned to the high rates that characterized the war years.

One of the key secondary goals of these chapters is to correct the erroneous periodization of twentieth century Cuba that prevails in most of the medical anthropology and public health literature. Uncritical use of the term "pre-revolutionary" obscures this dramatic variation in mortality patterns, and erases the importance of local and transnational variables in shaping these trends. The health and sanitation programs of the U.S. occupying army, for instance, contributed greatly to the turnaround in health conditions that followed the Spanish-Cuban-American War. Correspondingly, the rise in infectious disease that took place following the end of the U.S. military occupation appears to be more closely related to internal failures of Cuba's public health sector than to the increasing presence of North American capitalism on the island. Rather than blaming health problems during this time on "yankee imperialism" (as is common in Marxist scholarship), this historical research suggests that internal problems such as political corruption, *caudillismo* and political gangsterism destroyed the viability of public health programs during the republican years, and led to a resurgence of epidemic infectious diseases on the island.

Insight into the declines (and advances) in public health that occurred in Cuba during the republican years can be gained by examining the various kinds of activities necessary for effective control and prevention of infectious diseases. Even in the absence of a clinical or pharmaceutical cure, for instance, yellow fever and malaria can be prevented by strict mosquito control measures. Rates of typhoid and dysentery can be diminished by chlorinating water supplies, and tuberculosis deaths can be reduced by improving housing and nutrition.

Preventing diseases such as measles and smallpox requires compulsory inoculation. In other words, improving health conditions in any country requires many different kinds of activities, not just the importation of doctors and medical supplies. Engineers, entomologists, and vaccination specialists are also needed to control disease vectors at the source. In addition, there must be some sort of stable political authority in place to organize prevention campaigns and enforce health codes and quarantine laws.

Most of the Cuban governments between 1902 and 1959 did not respond effectively or appropriately to these public health challenges. During the republican era, political power in Cuba was most often seized by force, funds earmarked for public works improvements were freely appropriated by corrupt administrators, and health and education jobs were dispensed as sinecures, resulting in hugely overgrown government payrolls and inadequate attention to disease control. Public health sector employees were often expected to act as political partisans, selectively citing members of the opposition party for sanitary infractions, and excusing or ignoring infractions of political allies.

All of these factors increased health and sanitation problems throughout the country, as well as exacerbating the bitterness and violence of political opposition movements. This led to further insurrections, which exacted further costs on the physical infrastructure of the country. Political upheaval meant roads and transportation networks were destroyed, markets closed, commerce became paralyzed, public works projects were neglected, and agricultural production declined. These public sector failures destabilized the human environment in ways that facilitated outbreaks of infectious diseases.

Rethinking the State

What is the best way to theorize Cuba's violence, instability and public sector failures during the twentieth century? Orthodox Marxist scholars have typically blamed the inequalities and contradictions of capitalism, as well as the oppressive imperialism of the United States policies for these kinds of public health failures in Latin America and the Caribbean (see Navarro, 1976; Navarro, 1978; Taussig, 1974; Waitzkin, 1983; Waitzkin and Britt, 1989; Singer and Baer, 1989; Singer, Valentin, Baer and Zhongke, 1992).

U.S. political and military interventions in Cuba during the Platt era have typically been interpreted by leftist historians as a form of class struggle, with the imperial power of the United States assumed to act on behalf of U.S. capitalists eager to exploit Cuba's natural resources. Cuban political leaders from this time period are correspondingly viewed as compliant tools of the imperial power (or capitalist class) who facilitated the oppression of nationalistic Cubans (see Alarcón de Quesada, 1997; Castro, 1997a; Castro, 1997b; Instituto Cubano del Libro, 1973; Julien, 1968; Guevara Nuñez, 1997; Infante Marin, 1997; Leon Cotayo, 1997; Molina, 1997; Pino Santos, 1964; Rodriguez Alvarez, 1997; Benjamin, 1974; Blackburn, 1963; Pino-Santos, 1964; Simons, 1996).

My own research, however, suggests that a Weberian model of political capitalism offers more insight into the dynamics of Cuba's public health failures prior to 1959. Unlike Marx, Weber's approach to capitalism was focused on the variability of capitalist economies, and the way these variant forms result in very different kinds of political and economic structures. Weber iterated a number of different types, including "political capitalism," "modern industrial capitalism," "bourgeois capitalism," "colonial capitalism," "pariah capitalism," and "imperialist capitalism" among others (detailed in Gerth and Mills, 1958:49).

In Weber's model of political capitalism, politics and economic are configured in reverse from the conventional Marxist template. Rather than positing that political institutions emerge to serve the interests of capital, political capitalism involves having capital accumulation contingent on political connections. These dynamics have been described by Scott (1972:52) as follows,

> Politically oriented capitalism, whatever particular form it takes, involves the granting by the state of privileged opportunities for profit. Such openings are available only to those with connections or to those who can pay for influence. The "capitalists" in these circumstances are often officials inasmuch as state administrators are best placed to take advantage of the opportunities.

In a political-capitalist economy, there is no singular unified capitalist class. Instead, capital is divided into oppositional groups: the capital of political supporters of the regime, and that of political enemies. Personalistic armies and public officials are deployed to abet the capital accumulation of the loyal (who are often government officials), and to attack the capital of the opposition. In this sense, political capital-ism has much in common with the Latin American traditions of *caudillismo*, or strongman dictatorial government. In a *caudillo* state personalistic leaders use force to seize control of the public sector for private economic gain (see Andreski, 1966; Wolf and Hansen, 1966). One scholar has even referred to *caudillismo* as "a parasitic involution of capitalism" (Andreski, 1966).

Chapters 8 and 9 outline an alternative model of Cuba's twentieth century health history based on Weber's model of political capitalism. These chapters explore how Cuban leaders politicized large sections of the island's economy, and made capital accumulation in these sec-tors contingent on political support. In this model, the *polity* (or the government of Cuba) is viewed as a contested territory around which rival leaders (and their partisan armies) competed to gain control of the island's *economy*. In the Weberian model, capital does not suborn political leaders. Instead, political leaders use violence against one another to obtain the political power necessary to suborn or co-opt capital. In terms of health and disease, this model views the violence and destruction occasioned by these struggles, and the subsequent cor-ruption of the public sector for purposes of private profit, as leading to large scale failures in public health prevention efforts.

These aspects of Cuba's twentieth century history (violence, cor-ruption and *caudillismo*) have been described but not fully theorized by a number of contemporary historians (see Geyer, 1993; Langley, 1989; Thomas, 1998; Thomas, 2001; Perez, 1988; 1978; 1986; Suchlicki, 1969; 1997). Part of the problem lies in the constraints of language itself. To label certain behaviors (such as political payoffs or kickbacks) as "corrupt" implies they are intruding peripheral variables that contaminates a system but do not define it. In the case of Cuba prior to 1959, however, the behavior labeled "corruption" was often a defining feature of government itself.

To elaborate, in a political capitalist state, public officials use politi-cal power to extract rents or informal taxes on certain economic activi-ties. In return, businesses are granted political protections, such as favorable trading rights, freedom from competition, or monopoly privi-leges. As Scott (1972) has described,

Far from being pathological, patterns of corruption and violence may actu-ally represent channels of political demands without which formal societal arrangements could scarcely survive. . . . If the study of corruption teaches us anything at all, it teaches us not to take a political system or a particular regime at its face value. Corruption, after all, may be seen as an informal political system. . . . For most nations at some point in their history, and for many nations today, however, the surreptitious politics of this arena is so decisive that an analysis which ignored it would be not simply inaccurate but completely misleading. (1972:viii).

In the case of Cuba, understanding local patterns of corruption in the early twentieth century offers great insight into in the violence, instability and public health failures of the era. The bitter struggle for power that prevailed between rival political factions in the early years of the republic led each new leader to struggle for *political* control by seizing more *economic* resources. In this context, political power was used to restrict capital accumulation for those perceived as disloyal to the regime, and to enhance capital accumulation for political allies. Thus in the event of a "revolution" (a forcible takeover of the government by rebels), the wealth accumulated by political officials of the former regime would be immediately targeted for appropriation via looting or bureaucratic extortion.

The key argument of these historical chapters is that the violent factionalism of Cuban politics between 1902 and 1959 prevented the formation of a consistent, reliable public health sector capable of undertaking surveillance and vector control efforts necessary to prevent outbreaks of disease. Between 1902 and 1959, the "state" in Cuba was too contested, too parasitic, and too personalistic to coalesce into a viable authority that could enforce health codes and undertake crucial public works programs such as construction of water and sewer systems. By the early 1940s, advances in clinical medicine and medical technology in the *private* sector (such as the development of a vaccine to combat typhoid fever) helped control epidemic infectious diseases on the island, leading to a number of population health improvements. But *public* health (or government) prevention efforts, such as sewage treatment and proper chlorinating of drinking water, continually lagged due to the violence, instability and personalism of the political system. Further review of research in the political economy of corruption suggests that certain structural factors (particularly the inherent weaknesses and vulnerabilities of new states) seem to play a significant role in configuring the emergence of this pattern (see Scott, 1972; Tanzi,

1995; Rose-Ackerman, 1978; Wraith and Simkins, 1963; Zartman, 1995; Frimpong-Anash, 1992).

The United States and the Platt Amendment

The indigenous roots of Cuba's early political economy of corruption should not be taken to mean that the role of the United States in contributing to these problems was insignificant. The Platt Amendment, imposed on Cuba following the withdrawal of U.S. troops in 1902, meant that the United States necessarily became a major player in Cuban politics. The Platt Amendment granted the United States the right to intervene in Cuba in the event of political instability (or other conditions not to its liking), and also included an article (Article Five) specifically threatening intervention if Cuba failed to maintain appropriate health and sanitation programs.

These provisions in the Platt Amendment meant that between 1902 and 1933, no attempt to take power in Cuba could be successful without the implicit or explicit consent of the United States. This constraint led numerous Cuban political factions to form exile lobbying groups in the United States to petition the U.S. government *for* (not against) intervention under the Platt Amendment. The goal was to persuade the United States that the existing Cuban leader was violating the Constitution, jeopardizing the health and stability of the republic, and should be replaced with a new leader who truly embodied the will of the people. On several occasions, these campaigns were successful, and the United States intervened to engineer a change of power in Havana.

These efforts, however, typically resulted in little more than the substitution of one corrupt, unstable regime for another, as well as legitimate accusations of imperialism and increased tensions with other Latin American republics. When the United States refused to intervene in Cuba, however, the situation was hardly improved. Refusal to intervene led to charges that the United States was indirectly supporting a corrupt dictatorship by not acting aggressively to depose it.[4] If the United States appeared reluctant to intervene, opposition groups in Cuba would respond by shifting to increasingly violent tactics in an effort to bring the United States into the fray on their behalf. One of the most effective of these tactics was to threaten U.S. economic interests on the island by burning cane fields, with the hope that North

American businessmen would then pressure the United States to intervene. Thus the bitter factionalism of Cuban politics spilled over into the economy: threats of violence were used against foreign property as a means to politicize capital.

In other words, United States intervention in Cuba was not always done solely at the behest of U.S. economic interests, as Marxist scholars have assumed. U.S. interests were often diverse and contradictory due to the bifurcation of capital along political lines in Cuba, and the conflicting goals manifest between U.S. policy makers and U.S. capitalists. In some cases, U.S. businessmen actively joined forces with groups of Cuban insurgents, and together worked to manipulate U.S. political intervention (or nonintervention) under the Platt Amendment to their mutual (economic) advantage. Out of power factions frequently promised lucrative concessions to sympathetic businessmen in return for supporting a revolution or change of power in Havana. Lured by the thought of easy money, some of these business leaders supported Cuban insurgencies by supplying weapons to the rebels. In some cases, wealthy capitalists supported both sides in a political dispute to secure alliances regardless of the outcome of the rebellion.

Politicization of Health

In addition to facilitating instability in Cuba, the Platt Amendment also had important effects in the area of health and sanitation. Article Five of the Platt Amendment meant that health became a regular theme in the lobbying efforts of exile coalitions in their attempts to engineer support for U.S. intervention to overthrow the existing leadership in Havana. Out of power factions accused their rivals in Havana of allowing health and sanitation programs to lapse, thus endangering the fragile sovereignty of the new republic. Those in power, on the other hand, sharply denied these accusations and invoked nationalistic rhetoric against intervention. A number of Cuban leaders deliberately released false or misleading health reports to counter the accusations of exile coalitions in the United States. In other words, it is possible to find contradictory health statistics for nearly every Cuban administration from the early 1900s until the present. Official government health publications from the Platt era typically describe great progress in the control or eradication of infectious disease on the island. Exiled political opposition groups in Miami, Washington, DC, and New York, on the other hand, report widespread neglect of health and sanitation, as well as resurgent epidemic disease. These trends continued long after the abrogation of the Platt Amendment in 1933.

The politicization of health in Cuba during the Platt era makes it difficult to accurately chart health trends during this time. Official government reports and exile publications must be viewed with some degree of skepticism. Fortunately, there are alternative sources from which some idea of health trends in Cuba can be deduced. For the time period prior to 1959, these include internal Cuban health and sanitation reports, private correspondence from health officials, statistical reports from the United States Public Health Service station in Havana, journalistic reports (the *New York Times*, the *Dallas Morning News* and a number of other major U.S. newspapers maintained correspondents in Havana), diplomatic correspondence between Cuba and the United States, and reports by non-politicized agencies such as the Cuban Academy of Sciences.

These alternative sources suggest that nearly all of Cuba's political leaders prior to 1959 neglected health and sanitation programs to some extent during their years in power. In some cases (such as the regimes of Alfredo Zayas and Gerardo Machado in the 1920s), the effect of this sanitary neglect was especially negative. Epidemics of preventable waterborne diseases such as typhoid and enteritis swept through Havana regularly during the 1920s, killing thousands of people. Zayas borrowed millions of dollars from United States banks to fund construction of a new waterworks, but little or nothing was actually done to improve Havana's water supply. To deflect criticism from these activities, Zayas and Machado both released distorted health reports.

In other cases, this public health neglect was more benign. The second Batista regime (of the mid-1950s) was arguably as corrupt as that of Zayas in the 1920s, but by that point advances in clinical medicine such as antibiotics and vaccines were sufficient to control (though not prevent) outbreaks of infectious diseases. By the 1950s, international health agencies and North American newspapers were no longer reporting large-scale outbreaks of diseases such as typhoid and dysentery in Havana.

The Gangster-States

The Platt Amendment was abrogated in 1933, but Cuba's political factions remained bitterly divided. In 1933 a coalition of army sergeants and radical students overthrew the dictatorial Machado regime. This group immediately split into warring factions, who alternated their control of the government in Havana from the 1930s until the Castro revolution of 1959. Fulgecio Batista became the de facto leader of the army sergeants, and ruled from the 1930s until he was deposed in a national election in 1944. Batista later returned to power in a coup d'etat in 1952.

Batista alternated power with Dr. Grau San Martin, a professor at the University of Havana, and his followers. Grau was succeeded in office by his protégé, former anti-Machado student leader Carlos Prio Socarras. In general, the Grau/Prio groups were much more fragmented than the Batista faction, with some actively in favor of a formal alliance with the Soviet Union, and others taking an equally strong anti-communist position. Among the communists, there was also considerable tension between Trotsksyists and Stalinists, which led to violent conflicts. Only a few years after the 1933 revolution, there were at least seventeen radical leftist revolutionary groups fighting for power in Cuba, and inter-group shootouts, bombings and assassinations were common.

The various constituencies of the Grau and Prio regimes were united in their common desire to exploit the economic advantages of political office. Political power in Cuba became exponentially more lucrative during the 1920s, as the island became established as an offshore smuggling center for international criminal syndicates during Prohibition. As Scott (1972) has described, illicit capital is vulnerable to political extortion on a number of levels. Gangsters cannot conduct business without some degree of formal or informal cooperation by political authorities. This vulnerability led criminal syndicates to seek political protection from government officials in Cuba. In keeping with the traditions of political capitalism, favored racketeers were granted gambling and smuggling concessions, and politicians received a significant percentage of their earnings in return. Hugh Thomas (1998:1027), for instance, has estimated that in the 1950s, Batista and his followers received an estimated U.S. $1.28 million *per month* in payoffs from organized crime groups on the island. In some cases lucrative joint ventures were formed, and several Cuban politicians used their diplomatic credentials and immunity to smuggle narcotics to the United States on behalf of organized crime syndicates.

These dynamics led to a virtual fusion of organized crime groups with the formal political sector in Cuba by the end of the 1930s. These hybrid political-economic entities (which I have termed "gangster-states" or "racketeer-states") represent an elaboration of the earlier system of the political capitalist/*caudillo* system, but with the added (and volatile) variable of organized crime. In other words, the same politicization of capital that characterized the formal sector of the Cuban economy also characterized the informal sector. The use of personalistic security forces to secure monopoly rights for *caudillo*s and criminal syndicates, however, led to a parallel disenfranchisement of out-of-power political factions and aspiring racketeers, who often joined forces to try and topple the existing leadership in Havana. Unlike businessmen operating in the formal sector of the economy, racketeers maintain their own armies and weapons smuggling networks. As a result, there was a natural confluence of disenfranchised racketeers and out of power political coalitions. By the 1950s *economic* competition between rival racketeers in Cuba became increasingly intertwined with *political* competition between rival Cuban leaders. These dynamics were particularly apparent in the rebellion against the second Batista dictatorship (1952–1959) that ultimately brought Fidel Castro to power.

1959 and Beyond

Like many of his predecessors, Fidel Castro's regime has often mixed leftist ideology and gangster tactics. Sympathetic scholars in anthropology and public health frequently romanticize the former and ignore the latter while simultaneously emphasizing the gangster qualities of Castro's predecessors. This process effectively decontextualizes the Castro revolution from Cuba's long-standing historical traditions of *caudillismo* and violence. In reality, there are strong historical continuities between the Castro revolution of the late 1950s and earlier authoritarian regimes on the island.

Like generations of revolutionary groups before them, the 26 of July Movement was originally part of a much larger coalition organized by the deposed leaders of the previous regime. Together these groups initiated an aggressive lobbying campaign for the United States to intervene in Cuba to oust the existing leader. They also made strategic use of North American organized crime networks to procure weapons and supplies, and deliberately released distorted health data as a means to gain international support for their struggle.[5]

Once in power, the 1959 revolutionaries also reiterated many of the patterns manifest in earlier *caudillo* regimes. The original anti-Batista coalition soon became hopelessly fragmented, with some revolutionary leaders remaining with Castro in Havana, and others taking up arms against the new regime. The Castro government also engineered a complete changeover in the armed forces, imposed new state controls on vice and smuggling networks, increased militarization, established complete (and often personalistic) control over the island's economy, and disenfranchised dissidents or those perceived as disloyal to the regime. In these respects, the Castro government should be viewed as a logical successor to earlier *caudillo* regimes in Cuba.

There were also, however, a number of important changes and innovations that distinguished the Castro revolutionaries from their predecessors. From a public health point of view, one of the most significant of these was the substitution of a culture of civic honesty for the previous pattern of graft and corruption. The revolutionaries did eventually seize control of all productive enterprises in Cuba with the nationalization of the economy, but this governmental ownership was not solely for purposes of private enrichment as in earlier regimes. In the early years of the revolution funds earmarked for health improvements did reach their intended populations. Hospitals and health facilities were constructed in record numbers and aggressive prevention measures were put into place via neighborhood and community groups such as the CDR (Committees for the Defense of the Revolution) and ANAP (National Peasants Association). All of these activities certainly had favorable effects on health trends. The positive impact of political stability itself should also not be underestimated. The early years of the revolution saw a number of violent challenges to the Castro regime, but by the mid-1960s, all of the armed anti-Castro groups in Cuba had been virtually destroyed. Not counting the external forays of the Cuban military, the time period from 1963 to the present has been the most stable in Cuba's short history as an independent republic.

Recent evidence, however, suggests that many of these early positive trends have been reversed, especially since the fall of the Soviet Union in the early 1990s. A slew of scandals in the late 1980s and early 1990s suggest at least a partial return to the gangster-state politics of the 1950s.[6] A number of high-ranking Cuban officials have been implicated in activities such as money-laundering, narcotics smuggling and international prostitution rings in recent years. Health programs have lapsed, and many people prefer to seek treatment in the informal economy rather than the formal health system, due to the use of physicians as political informers. Increasing tourism and neglect of vector control efforts have also led to new problems with emerging infectious diseases on the island, such as dengue fever. If my own experience is any indication, the Cuban government is responding to these challenges with increased repression and denial rather than legitimate efforts to maintain favorable health conditions.

As long as foreign researchers and journalists are not allowed to undertake truly independent investigations on the island the truth about health conditions in Cuba since 1959 will remain unknown. At the very least, however, this work may help medical anthropologists and other researchers interested in the political economy of health to gain a more sophisticated understanding of Cuba that will help place these debates in proper historical context. For researchers interested in political economy of health in Latin America and the Caribbean, this work may offer the possibility of opening new possibilities for comparative research as well.'

Notes

1. I continued to follow Dr. Mendoza's case through *CubaNet News* after my return to the United States. At his trial in November, 1997 he was sentenced to eight years in prison for the crime of "disseminating counterrevolutionary propaganda." Following his sentencing, Amnesty International named him a prisoner of conscience and began a letter-writing campaign on his behalf. After serving one year in prison he was allowed to emigrate to the United States (Mendoza and Fuentes, 2001).

2. These included several collections the National Archives at College Park, Maryland, the Library of Congress, and the University of Miami and Emory University. In the spring of 1998 I also made a short return trip to Havana to do additional research in the National Library and the Carlos Finlay Museum. I also completed an exhaustive year-by-year review of the *New York Times* index to locate all relevant articles regarding health, disease and health politics in Cuba from the early 1900s through the early 1960s. Additional information was ob-

tained from back issues of the *Dallas Morning News* and the *New Orleans Times Picayune*—two newspapers that maintained active coverage of Cuban events during the early part of the twentieth century.

3. It should also be noted that this rejection of Marxism should not be taken as validation of the way Cuba has been portrayed by various anti-Castro extremists. A number of the assertions these individuals have made about Cuba can also be readily dismissed by a trip to the Island. The assumptions of the left, however, have become much more thoroughly embedded in academic discourse that those of the right. My critique thus focuses on challenging the portrayal of Cuba and the Cuban health care system by Marxist scholars.

4. The effects of both of these policy options of the Platt era (i.e., intervention or nonintervention) have been resoundingly criticized by contemporary scholars (see Benjamin, 1974; Benjamin, 1990; Perez, 1988; Perez, 1978; Perez, 1986; Paterson, 1994).

5. For discussion of former Cuban President Carlos Prio's early role in subsidizing the Castro revolutionaries, see Thomas, 1998. A good deal of information on Prio's activities (including arms smuggling) with the 26th of July Movement and other anti-Batista groups in the late 1950s can also be found in Prio's counterintelligence source files at the National Archives (RG 319). These records also detail a number of close relationships between anti-Batista factions and various organized crime figures in the United States.

6. For an overview of recent corruption and smuggling scandals in Cuba, see Oppenheimer (1993); Eckstein (1994); Corbett (2002); Morin (2003); Halperin (1994); Masetti (1993); Fernandez (1997).

Part One

The Ethnographic Encounter

1

Fieldwork

I first traveled to Cuba in the summer of 1995, full of curiosity and high hopes for my research project. This preliminary trip was immensely successful. Like many foreigners I fell deeply in love with the warmth and vitality of Cuba. All of the officials I spoke with seemed enthusiastic and supportive, and everyone (from university professors to random strangers on the street) seemed eager to talk about health. After three weeks of preliminary research, I returned to the United States and quickly convinced my dissertation committee that conducting long-term fieldwork in Cuba was a feasible research goal.

After completing my doctoral exams, I returned to the island in the winter of 1996, expecting to stay for at least a year of long-term fieldwork. The majority of the research was to be carried out in Santiago (Cuba's second largest city) located on the eastern end of the island. My visa was arranged through the University of the Oriente, and friends in Havana introduced me to an elderly widow in Santiago who would rent me a room. I liked Lydia[1] at once—she was warm and feisty and full of boisterous laughter. Her children lived in a neighboring province, and she continually told me how grateful she was to have some company in the house. I enjoyed her company too, and was very touched by her efforts to introduce me around the community and integrate me into her social world. By the end of January, 1997 I was comfortably settled and eager to begin my research.

The Field Site

The city of Santiago has always been quite different from Havana both culturally and geographically. It is older, less urbanized and moves at slower pace. One American observer in the 1920s in fact, described the cosmopolitan atmosphere of Havana as, "rather like Paris, a city of definite attraction where smart people go to be amused" (Woon, 1929:28). Santiago, on the other hand, was inevitably described as, "ancient," "retrogressive," "colonial." or "charming" (Terry, 1929; Woon, 1929).

In some ways these characterizations still hold true. Santiago remains a remarkably beautiful city, and *Orientales* (i.e., people from eastern Cuba) continue to define themselves as culturally distinct from Habaneros. The two regions, in fact, maintain stereotypes of each other somewhat reminiscent of those that prevail between people from the Deep South and people from the northeast in the United States. *Orientales* describe *Habaneros* as supercilious, overly concerned with fashion and appearances, and too hurried to properly enjoy life. *Habaneros* in turn characterize *Orientales* as slow, backwards, and forever prone to forgoing work or ambition in favor of eating well and sitting comfortably on their porches engaged in social visits and frivolous conversation.

The city itself has grown dramatically since the 1950s, but nearly all of this growth has taken place at the periphery. The historic urban core and the port area have remained unchanged practically since the colonial era, and traveling outward from the city center feels something like time travel. From the colonial downtown, the architecture gradually changes from traditional Spanish design to the American-influenced art deco of the early Republican period, to "modern" American-style suburbs built in the 1940s and 1950s, and finally to prefabricated socialist housing blocks of the present regime.

The first American-style suburb was constructed in Santiago was the neighborhood of Vista Allegre. This neighborhood was originally built to showcase the elaborate mansions of early sugar barons and other provincial elites at the beginning of the twentieth century. Today many of these houses have been taken over by the government for use as day care centers, provincial ministries and other government offices, or have been subdivided into apartments.

Beyond Vista Allegre are the more traditional 1950s style suburbs that represent the last (and most modern) phase of urban development in Santiago prior to the Revolution. The neighborhood of *Sueño,* for instance, was built in the late 1940s and early 1950s. These houses were designed by an American developer and are reminiscent of the low, one-story, postwar suburban housing commonplace in any southern U.S. city. Since this style of housing represents the last phase of construction from before the Revolution, the houses of *Sueño* are still viewed as "new" and "modern" and thus highly desirable (although they are in reality quite decrepit, having had little in the way of maintenance for the past forty years).

On the outermost edge of the city, about five miles from the city center are endless miles of low concrete apartment buildings divided into various districts named after either heroes of Cuban Independence or of the 1959 Revolution. The "Distrito José Marti," contains almost a quarter of Santiago's total population. These concrete-block and cement structures were constructed as part of the revolutionary plans for urban development and reflect the socialist aesthetic in architecture and urban planning.

Santiago Soundscape

The timeless rhythm of life in Santiago is most readily conveyed not with a visual overview of the city, but through a description of the soundscape. Unlike the traffic noise and bustle of Havana, Santiago still feels and sounds quite agrarian—people keep livestock in their patios to supplement their state rations. Even in the "modern" barrio where I lived, I always woke to the sound of squealing pigs and crowing roosters, the cries of street vendors and the slow clip-clop of their horse carts up and down the city streets.

One vendor in particular, always startled me out of sleep with his sharp morning cries of *"Perejil! Perejil*! [parsley]" It echoed through the neighborhood with surprising resonance. *"Perejil! Perejil*!" Further away I could barely make out a long, drawn out, almost agonizing cry of *"Caaaaaarrrrbbbooonn"* [charcoal]. (Upon hearing him, Lydia would always complain, *"Dios mio,* that's not a sales pitch, it's a lament!") And on a nearby street another vendor sang rhythmically over and over again, *"Ajo! Ajo un peso ajo*! ['garlic! for one peso, garlic!']."

These vendors passed through the barrio nearly every morning, yet for some reason, they seemed to walk primarily in the streets surrounding my house. This meant that although I could always hear them, it was many months before I saw them. Their cries floated around the neighborhood, seemingly disconnected from any corporeal beings, to the point where I began to imagine them as some sort of exotic tropical birdcalls. The sharp, resonant, *"Perejil perejil!"* the distant, anguished, *"Carbbooooonnn"* the languorous singsong, *"Ajo, ajo un peso ajo,"* repeated over and over, echoing across streets and over lawns, sometimes near, and other times only faintly discernible in the distance.

By mid-morning the outdoor sounds were often superseded by the rattle and clamor of the kitchen. The sharp hiss of the pressure cooker, the rhythmic pounding of garlic cloves in a wooden mortar and pestle, loud laughter accompanying the inevitable exchanges of gossip through kitchen windows. Lunch is still the biggest meal of the day in Santiago, and the lack of modern kitchen equipment means that the senior woman of the house must devote the better part of the morning to preparing a full *almuerzo*. Even minimal meals still require a significant time investment—rice and beans must be painstakingly picked through by hand, day after day, to remove tiny rocks, and most kitchen equipment is old and scarcely functional.

In the highly desirable and ultra modern house where I lived, for instance, the kitchen was equipped with a 1955 GE electric stove, a 1956 GE electric blender, a newly purchased Italian-made refrigerator (a recently retired 1955 GE model sat in the corner, converted into a storage cabinet). Of the original four burners on the electric stove, two were completely defunct, and of the remaining two, one had only the outermost rings of the heating element left, and the other worked only at the highest temperature setting. A portable kerosene stove sat on one counter and was often used in place of the deteriorating electric stove, or when there were power outages. The kerosene stove had to be used sparingly though, since kerosene was often unavailable. An ancient thermos sat in a central position on the countertop, holding the day's supply of coffee, flanked by two tiny chipped espresso cups that dated from the 1940s. The top to the thermos had long since disappeared and been replaced by an equally ancient piece of cork wrapped in an old rag.

The stifling heat of the afternoon made it impossible to avoid falling into a languorous siesta after lunch. In many ways, the siesta was my favorite part of the day. The heat rose up in waves from the pavement outside, and the little concrete house itself seemed to buckle and sway under the onslaught of the sun's rays. Lydia emitted seismic snores from the back bedroom, providing a soothing bass line to the percussive clatter of my ancient blue 1960s electric fan as it turned in its tiny arc of breeze. I lay in bed looking out at the little stone patio, breathing the hot afternoon air, listening to the steady metallic whir of the fan as drowsiness overtook me.

Often I would wake an hour or so later to hear a *visita* arrive. The custom of the formal social visit has eroded somewhat in Havana, but remains quite strong in Oriente. *Visitas* were so common during my time in Santiago, in fact, that I can scarcely remember a day without at least two (usually more) drop-in visitors. This was in addition to the regular, established presence of neighbors, who often ducked in and out of the house at will, either to watch the nightly television soap opera, or to simply to sit and talk during a lull in their daily chores. At times, entire days seemed to consist of little more than one long, endless (and often hilarious) conversation, punctuated by the gentle creak of the cane rocking chairs moving back and forth across the cool tile of the shaded front porch.

The exclusive use of rocking chairs (the heat makes upholstered furniture impractical), and the overwhelming emphasis on sociability, humor and conversation gave most afternoons a tranquil feel. Cuban-American writer Margarita Engle aptly described this sensation in her book *Singing to Cuba*,

> He led his mother to another rocking chair facing mine. Then he found one for himself, and looking around the room, I realized that rocking chairs were the only seats available. They were scattered all over the room, big, imposing rocking chairs. As I child I had always loved hammocks and rocking chairs. I had associated them with stability, with relaxation, pa-tience and a dreamy state of mind found only in the very young and the very old (Engle, 1993).

The "dreamy state of mind" Engle talks about is an apt description of the way these visits often passed. The sun-soaked quality of the late afternoon, the gentle motion of rocking chairs, and the ebb and flow of dialogue and laughter all combined to create a faraway sense of lassi-tude and repose. People spend hour after hour immersed in the gentle sway of rocking chairs and endless flows of conversation with little motive other than the simple pleasure of each other's company.

Often these conversations took on a delightful dreamlike quality themselves, as people reinvented their frustrations with bureaucracy and food shortages into wildly comic narratives of improvisation and derring-do. Over time I would come to think of these storytelling sessions as emblematic of the special magic I most admired in Cubans—the unique cultural alchemy whereby they were able to transform their daily ordeals of suffering and deprivation into shared laughter and wit. The line between comedy and tragedy is rarely absolute in any context, and Cubans seem to navigate this boundary with exceptional agility and skill.

At night, the world often took on a surreal quality since practically the entire city, without fail, watched the same television soap opera at nine, followed by the evening movie at ten. The spatial closeness of the houses, and the fact that doors and windows were often left open to catch whatever meager breeze might be available, meant that any pedestrian walking through the streets was confronted with the singularly unusual auditory sensation of hearing the same sound track emanating simultaneously (and at high volume) from every house on the street.

Ethnographic Vignette: Getting Oriented

Early one morning, shortly after my arrival in Santiago, I set out on my bicycle in search of the provincial Ministry of Health office hoping to track down a list of recent health statistics for my neighborhood. I had gotten directions from a neighbor, but still managed to get lost in the unmarked streets near the Moncada Barracks. Eventually I found myself at a side entrance of the provincial hospital, where I spied a man and a woman in white lab coats chatting in front of the door.

"Excuse me," I said hesitantly, pulling up to them on my bicycle. "Can you tell me where to find the local office of the Ministry of Public Health?"

"Oh look! Now what did I tell you?" the woman exclaimed to her friend, laughing. She was tall and had light coffee-colored skin. Her long hair was stylishly done in numerous tiny braids. The man she was with smiled sheepishly. "I told you," she repeated, giving him a playful tug on the sleeve. "And look at the beautiful bicycle!" she said in awe. "With *velocidades* [speeds] and everything And the color. . . . "
My 18-speed mountain bike (a glorious metallic purple) inevitably

became object of much jealous admiration wherever I stopped. It stood out from the bedraggled one-speed Chinese models that populated the streets of Santiago like a sleek Mercedes in a parking lot full of Yugos. They spent some moments remarking on the beauty of it. "And what's your name?" the woman with the braids asked me.

"Mary Katherine," I replied.

"Ah, Meryl! like Meryl Streep!" she seemed delighted. Meryl Streep is wildly popular in Cuba, the one American actress that all Cubans can instantly identify. The reasons for this are obscure.

"Well, not exactly, it's actually Mary, not Meryl—" I began, only to be interrupted.

"And with green eyes too!" the woman nodded knowingly to her friend. He seemed shy and reticent. "See! I told you." She said smugly to him, then turned to me again. "Meryl, do you drink wine?" she asked suddenly.

"Um, yes." I said hesitantly. I was beginning to wonder if I would ever find the Ministry of Health. The thought of reading through health statistics, though, suddenly seemed quite dull in comparison to the unexpected turns of this particular conversation.

"*Ai, pero mira Tomás*," she exclaimed again, shaking her head. "*Gente fina! Pero fina, te lo digo!*"

"*Gente Fina*" means literally "fine people" and is used generally to refer to those perceived as aristocratic. From the context, I inferred that a taste for wine together with having green eyes and a marvelous bicycle of *velocidades* were sufficient to classify me as "*gente fina.*"

"Ah, Meryl, you don't know how perfectly timed your arrival is, here on your lovely bicycle of *velocidades*," she said.

"Well, I'm very glad," I said back to them. "Although I don't quite understand why. And do you know where the Ministry of Health is?"

They laughed even harder. The man finally spoke. "You see . . . " he began, but trailed off. "It's just that I was telling Marisa . . . well, I've been out here explaining a terrible problem to her. I've been suffering so terribly. Oh, Meryl," he placed his hand on my arm, suddenly serious."Meryl, in my heart . . . in my heart," he stammered "In my heart, I feel all the pain of Christ on the cross . . . " He went on in this way for some time, describing deep emotional suffering with lyrical intensity, the way one might confide in a very intimate friend. I found myself awash in sympathy, in part out of sheer awe at the poetic way he chose to articulate his angst.

After a long, meandering preamble, I finally managed to deduce that his wife of seven years had recently been unfaithful to him, and he felt caught in a terrible dilemma. On the one hand, the rules of machismo demanded that he throw her out (and even give her a beating in the bargain). On the other hand, he very much wanted to forgive her and continue their relationship because he still loved her. He and Marisa, both doctors in the hospital and old friends from medical school, had stepped out for a moment to discuss what should be done. And Marisa had advised him to at least separate from his wife, but not to lose hope because at any moment someone new and wonderful could come into his life. It was at that moment that I pulled up on my marvelous shining bicycle of *velocidades*—seeming proof of Marisa's prophecy.

After such a propitious introduction, I felt it would hardly be polite of me to simply demand directions to the Ministry of Health and leave. We spent the better part of an hour standing by the back door of the hospital, suddenly immersed in an entirely unexpected and intimate sociality, something that I would soon come to realize was a uniquely Cuban experience.

As they prepared to go back into work, Marisa told me to come by her house the following afternoon and she would take me to the Ministry of Health herself, and introduce me to a friend of hers who worked there. Feeling a little overwhelmed at having my afternoon plans completely reconfigured by this chance encounter, I agreed.

Knowing the casual attitudes most Cubans kept about punctuality, I showed up at Marisa's house at 2:30 P.M. the following afternoon. Unfortunately, I had still underestimated the appropriate degree of lateness for such an appointment. Marisa groggily answered the door in her threadbare *bata de casa* (the loose, cotton housedresses most Cuban women wear inside), obviously in the middle of her siesta. She gestured for me to sit on the couch and retreated to her bedroom to change. The house was a ramshackle affair, with ancient, threadbare furniture. A pile of bricks sat in the middle of the living room, someday to be used to build an additional room. At present there were nine extended family members sharing the house, which was headed by Marisa's mother and maternal uncle (a matrilineal arrangement I would later come to realize is quite common in Cuba).

It was over an hour later before we finally set out for the Ministry of Health, and many more hours before we finally arrived. The office was only about a ten minute walk from Marisa's house, but she insisted on taking me first to a small food stall near the hospital to introduce me to her mother, where we spent some time in conversation, and then to a cousin's house for coffee and yet another long, conversational visit. We finally got to the Ministry of Health around 4:00 P.M. What had begun as a simple request for directions had turned into a full day of social visits, guided tours of the city and informal interviews. At the time I was quite amazed to find my research agenda so abruptly hijacked by well-meaning strangers. Eventually though, being led on such epic adventures by total strangers in response to simple requests for information began to feel quite normal. While it did wreak havoc with my (heretofore carefully planned) research agenda, I eventually grew to embrace the sheer chaotic Cuban-ness of it.

Note

1. Unless otherwise indicated, all names and other identifying information have been changed. In some cases even genders and localities have been disguised to prevent retribution against Cubans who spoke openly with me.

2

Doing Research, Not Doing Research

Like many research proposals, mine looked good on paper, but proved to be utterly unworkable once I got to the field. In one of my first meetings with the Director of International relations at the University of the Oriente (my official sponsor) I was informed that I would not be allowed to use any questionnaires or survey instruments, and that each phase of my project had to be approved and supervised by at least two members of the faculty. Any requests for information had to be mediated by my supervisors at the university. They would also require me to pay them a substantial research fee in American dollars. Given my meager resources, and (in my opinion) the outrageousness of the monetary request I became somewhat resentful. As a compromise I offered to pay them month-by-month. It put a serious dent in my finances, but I was in no position to argue.

At that point, I should have been able to leap wholeheartedly into the research—interviewing doctors, following up patients, getting to know people in the community and participating as much as possible in everyday life. Unfortunately, this was not the case. People were friendly, but resistant to formal queries for information. It seemed like I got nowhere as an anthropologist, trying to do the things that anthropologists are supposed to do. People stood me up for interviews and blew off meetings. One doctor said I needed permission from the Ministry of Health before I could visit his clinic. Another said I needed a written letter of introduction from the University of the Oriente. A third said I needed permission from his supervisor in the local health department. There was no consensus as to what bureaucratic channels I should pursue to get access to the information I needed. It was all intensely frustrating and very time consuming. I spent hours sitting in offices waiting for various bureaucratic approvals, which invariable never came. On the few occasions health professionals did agree to be interviewed they seemed to limit themselves to polite trivialities.

My supervisors at the University of the Oriente responded to my pleas for help with complete indifference. Often I would schedule meetings to ask for advice and no one would show up. This occasioned some sympathy from friends and neighbors, several of whom implied that such behavior on the part of University officials towards foreign students was not unknown.

"There was a group of Canadians who came here to study Spanish," one friendly professor remarked with a wry grin. "The University made them pay in cash, up front for their classes. Then they kept postponing the classes until the students' visas ran out and they had to leave. You were smart to offer to pay them month by month," he added. "If you had given them all your money at the beginning I doubt you would have heard from them again."

Another friend spoke even more bluntly, "Dr. [Supervisor]?" He laughed. "Be careful with him. He's a gangster. In it up to his eyeballs with [other higher ups]. For sure they're splitting the money amongst themselves. He'll be using it to build a raft and sail to Miami, just like all the rest. Pay him month-by-month—as little as possible. It's the only way you'll keep him on his toes." Two Canadian students told me the same thing: they had paid the university in advance for classes in Spanish literature but the classes never happened. The students decided to just hang around Santiago, listening to local music groups and drinking beer until their money ran out.

Around this time I began keeping a field diary. The first entry reads rather bleakly as follows:

I am beginning this diary in the depths of despair. I have now been in Cuba two full months and feel like I have accomplished nothing. I am met at every turn by smiling, friendly faces who welcome me with great enthusiasm only to nod sadly and refer me back to the same faceless bureaucracy—cold, endless, timeless and utterly without remorse—when I try to amplify the contact.

Informal Research Methods

But before long (as is the case in all troubled fieldwork narratives) things began to change. It dawned on me gradually: the key to doing good anthropological fieldwork in Cuba, it seemed, was to avoid being an anthropologist. When I tried to do what anthropologists are supposed to do (asking people behind desks for information or formal interviews) I got nowhere. But when I was interacting with people socially, off the record, they seemed quite willing to talk at length and freely answered all of my questions. As long as my requests were informal and mediated through my broadening (fictive) kin and social networks, I had no trouble with access. If I tried a formal request, mediated through my official sponsors at the university, I got nowhere.

When I puzzled over this inconsistency out loud to friends and neighbors they laughed at my naiveté. Apparently the formal bureaucratic system in Cuba was viewed as so unwieldy and complex that everyone tried to avoid going through formal channels at all whenever possible. Instead, they explained, people worked informally, using personal networks of friends and relatives with whom they exchanged favors to accomplish bureaucratic (or other) goals. These individuals were termed "*socios*" ("friends"), and people jokingly used the term "*sociolismo*" to describe the lived reality of their socialist system.

It certainly wasn't hard to see examples of *sociolismo* in action all around me. One neighbor complained about the chore of cultivating a personal relationship with an individual in the Ministry of Education in order to get her daughter placed in a desirable school. Another described participating in an elaborate network of economic barter that involved trading sheets and towels (stolen from a local tourist hotel) for soap and kerosene (stolen from a state supply warehouse). Commodities obtained this way were often traded for food with vendors who traveled to the city from outlying rural areas carrying clandestine packages of chickens, eggs, fish or meat. "Everyone does it [steals from the state]," he said with a twinkle in his eye. "It's the only way to survive." There seemed to be no moral stigma attached to this kind of behavior. In fact, people who were exceptionally clever in their pilfering were often admired in the community and awarded great cultural caché.

It was easy to see the motivation for stealing or trading on the black market—the standard monthly ration of food for a single household would barely last two weeks, leaving a significant period of time in which food had to be borrowed, hustled, bought on the black market or purchased in the wildly overpriced dollar stores. A strong network of *socios* could mean the difference between going hungry and finding enough to eat. In bureaucratic terms, well-placed *socios* could also improve life in other important ways—engineering a transfer from a run-down hospital with limited running water and no medical supplies to a well-stocked, elite clinic. *Socios* could also be used to arrange for more desirable housing, transportation and jobs. Everyone seemed to agree, life without *socios* would be virtually impossible in Cuba.[1]

This realization posed an interesting research problem. If I tried to be a "good" anthropologist and follow the rules my research sponsors had set for me (i.e., requesting information only through formal channels) most likely I would spend the remainder of my time in Cuba in the grips of paralyzing bureaucratic inertia, scheduling endless meetings at which no one showed up, and ultimately accomplishing none of my goals. Any data I did obtain via official channels would also be unreliable, since I had already discovered that few people were willing to voice honest opinions in the context of a formal interview. One friend confirmed my suspicions by stating, "We know we're supposed to be moving toward democratic reforms and be able to speak out, to criticize. But people are still scared. Any kind of survey or opinion poll makes them afraid. No one will say what they really think." Under such conditions, it seemed as if following proper methodological procedures would result in highly compromised data.

On the other hand, if I used informal contacts and informal methods I could obtain more honest information but my research would be ethically and methodologically questionable. Essentially I would be violating the terms of my agreement with the University of the Oriente, as well as the informed consent protocol of the Emory University Institutional Review Board. It was a troubling dilemma: should I follow proper procedures even if it meant obtaining compromised data? Or should I make the effort to get honest information even if it meant bending some of the standard ethical practices for anthropological fieldwork?

Intellectual curiosity ultimately won out. The ethics of not strictly following consent protocols troubled me greatly (and still do), but it was too maddening to be there, to have the answers to my research questions so close at hand, and not be able to pursue them. Plus by that point I was beginning to suspect an entire generation of medical anthropologists had been seriously mislead about the nature of the Cuban health care system precisely because they had not been able to conduct true ethnographic fieldwork in Cuba. The comments people made to me informally about health and health care were radically different from the descriptions I had read of the Cuban health care system in the scholarly literature.

I decided to stay and learn as much as I could, even if it meant working informally. There was no way I was going to allow my research to grind to a bureaucratic halt or to be misdirected by the distortions of official interviews. And besides, I rationalized, if it was local custom to circumvent bureaucracy and work via informal channels, an argument could be made that I was simply adjusting my plan to reflect local norms—something anthropologists are supposed to do in the field. While methodological rigor is lost in this approach, informal research does have some significant advantages.

Anthropologists who study criminal subcultures in the United States, for instance, frequently use informal methods since few people are willing to speak openly or honestly about taboo or illegal behavior. Ferrell (1998) has used the Weberian term "verstehen" to describe the advantages of trading the objectivity of statistical or survey methods for subjective personal experience with the culture or subculture under study,

> As formulated by Max Weber and developed by later theorists, *verstehen* denotes a process of subjective interpretation on the part of the social researcher, a degree of sympathetic understanding between social research and subjects of study, whereby the researcher comes to share, in part, the situated meanings and experiences of those under scrutiny (Ferrell, 1998:27).

The goal of this approach is to trade the tools of objective research for personal risk and immersion, entering as completely as possible into the life worlds of their informants in order to "feel and understand the situated logic and emotion" of the environment (Ferrell, 1998:28). Informal methods can also "reveal parts of the social world that remain hidden by more traditional techniques" such as surveys and interviews (Ferrell, 1998:24). Safely distanced methods like questionnaires cannot approach key issues of subjectivity or emotion; pain or pleasure—areas that (Ferrell argues) are crucial in apprehending the "lived experience" and "situated emotions" of individuals. Other researchers have described this strategy as taking on a "membership role,"

> The advantage of taking a membership role over other forms of research involvement lies in members' recognition of the researcher as a fellow member. This allows the researcher to participate in the routine practices of members, as one of them, to naturalistically experience the members' world. Doing "membership work" forces the researcher to take on the obligations and liabilities of members. In repeatedly dealing with the practical problems members face, researchers ultimately organize their behavior and form constructs about the setting's everyday reality in much the same way as members. . . . A final advantage of taking on a membership role is that researchers can gain access to "secret" information. This information, known only to members, ratifies the solidarity and continued existence of the group (Adler and Adler, 1987).

For me, taking on a membership role in Cuba meant I had to surrender my identity as a researcher and learn local norms of social behavior. My role in Lydia's household ceased to be one of a visiting professional or outsider and instead became a more personal role of adopted daughter. This meant I gradually became incorporated into her extended social and kin network. Given the very close ties Cubans typically maintain with their friends and families, I was soon enmeshed in a close-knit social circle. I found these relationships to be tremendously rewarding—I was often overwhelmed with the warmth and hospitality of Cuban social life, and came to appreciate the idyllic portrayals of Cuban society so common in exile literature.

A major disadvantage of using informal research methods, however, was that it meant I became constrained by local norms governing the behavior of young, unmarried women. Proper Cuban daughters are not supposed to venture out alone on the streets—to do so is viewed as unseemly, as it invites aggressive male attention. One day in Havana I observed a seventeen year old girl I knew standing outside the front door sharing a joke with the man who delivered the bread in the afternoons. He grandfather became furious with her. "*Que putaría!* [what whorishness!]" he shouted at her as she walked back into the house. She later told me her brother had reacted in a similar fashion when he saw her talking with some (male) schoolmates in the street one day. He had insisted she return home with him immediately.

These kinds of restrictions on women were by no means universal, but as Mona Rosendahl has described, Mediterranean gender norms continue to shape the behavior of men and women in Cuba, despite considerable revolutionary rhetoric to the contrary,

> Traditional attitudes regarding gender issues are still prevalent among both men and women [in Cuba], which makes gender equality rather limited in everyday life. In reality, there is both gender stratification and a gendered division of labor. Men have most of the power in Cuban society. . . . The gender system in . . . most parts of Cuba, is based on an inheritance of Mediterranean and Caribbean views of gender. . . . Virginity, motherhood, and chastity are important female traits, while the male is seen as the protector of and provider for his family, as well as a virile lover (Rosendahl, 1997:52–53).

These sentiments were also expressed somewhat more bluntly by Carlos Alberto Montaner, who stated, "[T]he Cuban Revolution is covered by a layer of hairy machismo" (1981:143).

In Santiago, young women who do venture out of the house alone are supposed to show proper decorum: they should not respond to *piropos* (suggestive comments men make to them on the street) initiate conversations with strangers, or invite strangers over to the house. Unfortunately, all of these activities are necessary for good anthropological fieldwork. These gender norms were never formally spelled out for me—no one ever deliberately sought to restrict my movements or activities. But in the course of everyday conversations with Lydia and her family it became clear that daughters and "good" women were expected to behave this way.

Several of Lydia's neighbors tried to earn extra money by renting out rooms to tourists, for instance, and often came over to share their shock and horror at the way single men would bring *jiniteras* or prostitutes into their homes. Such women were spoken of in very disparaging terms, and their presence in a "respectable" house was most unwelcome. One neighbor viewed these women as so polluting that she obsessively disinfected her entire house after such a visit, and even described pulling the tourists' sheets off of the bed with a broomstick so she wouldn't have to touch them.

Personally I was very interested to know more about the lives and experiences of Cuban prostitutes. Fidel Castro had once boasted that Cuba had "the best educated prostitutes in the world" since so many highly educated women were now "*jiniteando*" due to the economic crisis. These developments were inevitably portrayed by foreign journalists as representing either great moral decline, admirable entrepreneurship or tragic female despair. I was curious to know how the *jiniteras* themselves felt about their behavior. Was it true they could earn as much in a single night as a surgeon earned in a month? Did they feel that had status in the new Cuba as major breadwinners for their families? Or did they feel stigmatized?

In my symbolic role as a daughter in Lydia's house, there was no way I could interact socially with *jiniteras*. They were inevitably described by the senior women in my neighborhood as low, dirty, carriers of disease and representative of an "undesirable element." If I were to interact with *jiniteras* (especially if I were to bring them into Lydia's home) I would symbolically contaminate and scandalize myself to the point where I would no longer be viewed as socially acceptable by the women in the neighborhood. While I was sure they would still be kind and polite to me, I would lose my insider access among that particular group.

Listening to neighborhood women speak disparagingly of the *jiniteras* also made it clear that Cuba, despite years of egalitarian rhetoric, still maintains a number of sharp social divisions. The neighborhood where I lived, for instance, was relatively elite. Nearly all of the people on my street were light-skinned, had connections to the communist party (or other powerful revolutionary credentials), as well as relatives in Miami to send them extra money.

A number of houses sported such luxuries as color televisions, VCRs, telephones, cars, or washing machines. Some even had the most coveted item of all—a window air conditioning unit. Many of the families had lived in the neighborhood since before the Revolution, meaning they were pre-revolutionary elites. Others had acquired their desirable houses as rewards from the revolutionary government itself. One house on the block was newly occupied by *a jinitera,* whose wealthy Italian boyfriend had purchased it for her.[2] But the other women in my social circle refused to have any contact with her.

Blacks ("*los negros*") were also looked down on by my network of *socios.* Many neighbors warned me that if I walked around Santiago by myself carrying a camera (which I often did) "*los negros*" would surely rob me. Others gave me even more dire warnings: "*los negros*" would steal my bicycle, assault me, and take everything from the house if I were to leave it unattended for even a moment. One day I witnessed a neighborhood grandmother berate her daughter for letting her eight year old walk across the street alone: "You let your daughter walk around unaccompanied with the quantity of *negros* that pass through this neighborhood!" she admonished.

These prejudices and social divisions placed onerous limits on my activities. Unlike my neighbors, I did not fear "*los negros*" and would have liked to talked to people of as many different backgrounds as possible. After witnessing these kinds of exchanges, however, I felt that attempting to broaden my social network to include people of different backgrounds would cost me a lot of rapport with Lydia and her circle. Given how kinship ties still seemed to structure most social interactions in Santiago, it seemed wiser to maintain the integrity of my membership role even if it meant sacrificing diversity of opinion in my research.

Despite these restrictions I did manage to accomplish some of my research goals, albeit in a more restricted way than I had first envisioned. My network of *socios* gradually expanded to include several local physicians, who graciously agreed to allow me to come and visit their clinics. These doctors in turn introduced me to other health professionals who spoke with me informally about practicing medicine in Cuba. Eventually I managed to conduct approximately fifty hours of informal clinic observations in four different family doctor clinics in Santiago. In addition, these observations were supplemented by approximately twenty-five informal interviews with physicians in their homes. Additional informal interviews were also conducted with other health professionals, including nurses, dentists, social workers, and three professionals at the University of the Oriente. I also attended a health economics conference sponsored by the local medical school that provided useful data on the economic dimension of local health services. Considerable time was also spent conducting archival research at the University of the Oriente library, the provincial archives and the medical school library.

During my time in Santiago, friends and neighbors also took great pains to instill another troubling restriction: I should never discuss my political beliefs. "Never talk politics with anyone," was a whispered warning I heard on at least six different occasions. "Like if someone comes up to you on a bus or on the street and starts a conversation. Just avoid it altogether. Don't say anything." I was still rather naive at the time, but savvy enough to grasp what they were implying: the state security (a force that inspired such fear it was never spoken of out loud) might try to elicit uncensored political opinions from me in the guise of casual conversation. If I were foolish enough to speak openly to them or criticize the Cuban system, it could have very negative consequences.

I intuited early on that such subjects were deeply taboo, and was always careful to avoid making any negative or critical remarks about the Cuban government. Again, to my surprise, people often seemed quite willing to express dissatisfaction and dissent to me, sometimes in remarkably forthright language. Phrases such as "This system is shit," "There is no freedom here," "The repression is worse now than it has ever been," and "The health care system is *jodido*" [polite translation: the health care system is really screwed up] were not uncommon. Irreverent jokes and comments about *El Líder Maximo*[3] were also frequent occurrences. Televised political speeches invariable occasioned sighs of exasperation, or an occasional muttered, "When is this guy going to shut up?" Others cloaked their dissatisfaction in more abstract terms, and it was not uncommon to hear people make vague statements about "the evils of politics." They were always careful not to specify what or who's politics they were talking about, but it was clear by the tone they used these were not idle speculations.

These conversations instilled a moderate degree of paranoia in me as I began to understand more about Cuba. By opting out of a formal researcher role and into a membership role, I had become privy to expressions of political dissent and dissatisfaction that people would probably not have voiced under other circumstances. Revealing my awareness at the widespread political dissent, however, would have been impossible. There was no way I could initiate a conversation by saying, "Your neighbor Fulano said he thinks the government is repressive and hopelessly corrupt. Do you agree?" Instead I had to go about my daily life and informal research as if I were still blissfully ignorant of these sentiments. As my awareness of the dissent and dissatisfaction that circulated in the community increased, it became increasingly difficult to maintain this facade.

It was also worrisome to realize just how uncritical previous medical anthropologists and public health researchers had been in their assessments of Cuba and the Cuban health care system. The gap between the way social scientists have described revolutionary Cuba and the way the people in my community in Santiago seemed to feel about their political system, and the role of the health care system in the context of socialism was profound. I had brought a large packet of academic journal articles on Cuba with me to the field. Each was singularly laudatory in its own way. "I left with a strong sense of respect," one Canadian physician exclaimed. Others marveled at how the Cuban Revolution had "improved and humanized" health care (see Waitzkin and Britt, 1989; Wald, 1978; A. Chomsky, 2000).

In one sense, these assertions were true. Cuba had equalized access to health care since the Revolution. They had developed a number of innovative primary care programs. They had equalized income across all sectors of the population, subsidized food and improved nutrition. According to MINISAP statistics, all of these programs together had profoundly positive benefits for the health of the Cuban people: infectious diseases that continued to plague neighboring countries had been virtually eliminated in Cuba. All of these were laudable achievements.

Nonetheless, after living in Santiago for several months, I couldn't help but feel these previous researchers had missed something important. There seemed to be a considerable gap between the way Cuba was portrayed by North American medical anthropologists and public health researchers, and the way Cubans themselves described their system in informal speech. These previous researchers had either overlooked the cynicism and mistrust I kept encountering, or else they had chosen to ignore it. Given how pervasive these sentiments were in my everyday experience, however, I could not bring myself to ignore them. One of the most fundamental goals of ethnographic research is to get "the native's point of view." In my case the natives often seemed powerfully disenchanted with their system in ways that North American academics were not.

This discrepancy intrigued me and I maintained something of a dual research strategy over the succeeding months. I continued my clinic observations and informal contacts with doctors and nurses, while at the same time keeping my ears open for expressions of criticism or discontent. I couldn't formally initiate such discussions, but I could gently probe if people informally volunteered information or anecdotes. Given the almost total exclusion of North American researchers from long-term participation in Cuban communities over the past forty years, it didn't seem too unreasonable that the Cubans might know something that medical anthropologists did not.

Notes

1. For an excellent analysis of Cuba's informal economy and economic illegalities on the island in the Special Period, see Henken (2005) and Ritter (2005). For a more general discussion of economic illegalities and morality in Cuba see Morin (2003).
2. Since the government owns all housing it is technically illegal to buy and sell residential property in Cuba. These rules are circumvented in a variety of creative ways.
3. No one in Cuba ever refers to Fidel Castro by name. Instead a variety of colorful euphemisms are used such as "your crazy uncle," (as in, "You won't believe what your crazy uncle has done now.") For an especially critical remark, a Cuban might simply brush his cheek with his finger or make similar gesture pantomiming a beard.

3

Dengue Fever: An Abrupt
Change of Perspective

Rumors of an outbreak of dengue in Santiago began circulating as early as February of 1997. The little old ladies in my exercise class murmured nervously amongst themselves every time a mosquito happened by. Still, there was no official word and few people appeared overtly concerned.

In April I noted with some curiosity a small article in *Granma* that mentioned an increase in the presence of the *Aedes aegypti* mosquito (the mosquito that carried dengue) in Oriente province (April 17, 1997). The article took pains to assure readers that the mosquito was "familiar" and "inoffensive" and that dengue had been completely eradicated in Cuba in 1981 (*Granma*, April, 17, 1997). Given the persistent rumors of a dengue outbreak, I felt sufficiently intrigued by this article to clip it from the newspaper and put it in a file of other health-related clippings.

Several weeks later I attended a health economics conference organized by the medical school in Santiago. The conference was particularly important for me since much of the data that was to be presented (information on hospital occupancy rates, policlinic visits, infectious disease and patient care) was exactly the same information that the provincial ministry of health had been refusing to release to me for several months.

By the middle of the first day of the conference I was overcome with tremendous fatigue and sore throat, but wrote it off as a combination of stress, undernourishment and the extreme air-conditioning of the conference center. Lydia had gone to Havana to visit her family the previous week, and my diet had suffered accordingly—there was almost no food that could be purchased anywhere near the house or conference center (even for dollars), and there was little in the way of state rations distributed that month.

By the third day of the conference, I began to suspect something more serious than worry and fatigue might be wrong with me. The closing panel was devoted to detailing all of the negative effects of the U.S. embargo on Cuba's health care system. The final speaker concluded his remarks with a long speech implying that the United States was deliberately trying to resist academic exchanges with Cuba because they didn't want Americans to learn of Cuba's scientific advancements and health achievements. Hearing these accusations, after months of obfuscation from the local health office, threw me into such a snit that I was determined to speak to him after the lecture. But then, as I tried to stand up and walk to the front of the room, my knees buckled abruptly and I nearly collapsed. After a few moments my head stopped spinning and I recovered enough to walk, but the extent of my weakness and fatigue was becoming worrisome.

Later that evening I mentioned to a friend that I had been feeling sick, and wondered if I might have contracted hepatitis.

"Be careful you don't get dengue," he warned me gravely. "It's all over the city now, and they say the hospitals are getting full and five or six people have died."

"Dengue!" I exclaimed. "But I haven't seen anything in the papers. Why haven't they publicized it? Anyway, I don't think I'm sick enough to have dengue. I'm sure it's just a virus or something. Maybe hepatitis, but not dengue."

"Just be careful," he cautioned me. "And go to the doctor if you have any fever."

The next day I went to continue my observations in one of the family doctor clinics I had been working with. During a lull between patients I mentioned that I had been feeling sick. She immediately looked alarmed.

"Have you had any fever?" she asked.

"No, not really," I said. "I've mostly felt chilled, like with a virus. I've been so weak and tired, I was thinking it might be hepatitis or something, but then someone mentioned that there was an outbreak of dengue. Is that right? Is there dengue?"

She looked momentarily frightened. "No . . . no there's no dengue," she said slowly. "But there is this virus going around that has some similarities to dengue. So don't hesitate to come back if you have any fever or anything. You know we'll take good care of you," she smiled weakly.

I took several days off to recuperate, and my condition improved somewhat. The flu symptoms dissipated and only the fatigue remained. I managed to convince myself that I wasn't really sick, and that it was the emotional stress of fieldwork that was causing me to lapse into a Malinowskian hypochondria. Having read Malinowski's published field diary (which obsessively details every little physical ailment that afflicted him) before I left for Cuba, I was determined not to make such a spectacle of myself. The cure for my malaise, I decided abruptly, would be just to work. Given my limited improvement, it seemed silly to worry about being afflicted with a disease as serious as dengue. I had known a woman in Ecuador who had dengue and said it was one of the most intensely painful and debilitating things she had ever experienced. I dismissed my fatigue and sore throat as trivial somatizations.

The next morning, just as I was washing up the breakfast dishes, I was hailed over the patio wall by an elderly neighbor. "Katherine!" he barked, charging up to the side door waving the rusty old machete he used to trim the lawn. I could tell by the expression on his face I had done something to displease him.

"*Estoy muy bravo contigo,*" he lectured me sternly in his staccato Spanish. "Lourdes told me you were sick, but you didn't you tell me you needed help! You know Lydia left us in charge of you. And you went and got sick because you don't eat right—look how skinny you're getting—" he poked me in the ribs with the point of his machete, "—and you still won't ask us to bring you anything. Well today, *mijita,*" he said accusingly, "my wife is making you a big pot of soup and you're going to eat. When you get ready for lunch you yell over that patio wall and we'll put on some rice for you—"

"But Fernandez," I protested meekly, "I wasn't very sick, really. I'm much better now, and I hate to be a bother—"

He glared at me until I fell silent. A retired military officer, Fernandez tended to speak in commands, rather than sentences. And I could tell I had deeply offended him by failing to ask for his help when I wasn't feeling well. All of the neighbors had tried to help out while Lydia was away by bringing me food and repeatedly lecturing me that I should never hesitate to ask for something if I needed it. At first I had assumed these offers were motivated by sincere intentions, but that food was so scarce that it would be wrong of me to take more than a token offering. Fernandez' anger, though, made me realize that my attitude made me appear to be holding myself aloof from the deep ties of reciprocity that held this group of individuals together.

Throughout my first few months in Santiago, I had freely dispensed band-aids, aspirin, cough drops, antibiotic cream and English lessons to a steady stream of shy but needy neighbors. Now that I was in need, however, I had refused to allow them to return the favors they had incurred. In Cuba, such one-sided generosity is viewed with considerable hostility, as it implies a certain snobbishness and flaunting of wealth. I had once heard one neighbor criticizing her daughter-in-law for being too "*auto-suficiente*" (self-sufficient), and belatedly realized that asking for help was a vitally important step for me to take if I wanted to be treated as an equal in this social world. Meekly, I told Fernandez that I would spend the whole day resting and eating to try and get my strength back.

"Be sure that you do," he commanded. I smiled inwardly at the irony of being forced into a Malinowskian hypochondria the sake of my fieldwork after all.

Oddly enough, as the day progressed I found myself feeling sicker and sicker. The weakness and fatigue returned, along with severe joint pains and a dull ache behind my eyes. The sunlight seemed painfully bright, as if I were in the early stages of a migraine.

"Katherine, I heard you weren't feeling well." One of the doctors I had been working with stopped by for a visit.

"Word travels fast," I smiled, rolling my eyes.

She laughed. "You know, around here everybody knows everything about everybody. Let me tell you, there are no secrets in this town."

I laughed with her. "It's true. I mentioned to one neighbor yesterday that I wasn't feeling well, and already I've had two pots of soup brought over and three visitors to check on me. Santiago is a big city, but it feels like a small town."

"Yes, that's why I like it better than Havana," she agreed. "But tell me, really, how are you?"

"I was sick for a few days, but I don't think it's anything serious. I'm still really tired though. I'm sure I'll be fine."

"No fever or anything?"

"No, no just chills, like with a virus."

"Okay," she said maternally, "but if any of the symptoms come back, please come and see me. Don't be *auto-suficiente*," she warned.

A few hours later a public health nurse came by, canvassing the neighborhood for anyone with fever, weakness, fatigue, aches or diarrhea. When I told her I had had all of these things she ordered me to report to my family doctor's in the morning.

"But why—?" I began, but she was already walking away, up the sidewalk to Ferndandez' house.

Dengue

Other visitors came and went as the day passed. My headache continued to worsen. At six o'clock I moved my rocking chair inside, took one of my carefully hoarded codeine pills, turned out the lights and went to bed. Lying in darkness eased the sharpness in my eyes, but the headache expanded dramatically to encompass my entire skull. Nothing helped. I lay in bed, hunched and tiny and still, able only to breathe, while the pain circled through my head in wild burning spirals.

I remember at some point in the night I tried to get up and find my way to the bathroom. I held on to the wall, but sank to my knees, unable to see or keep myself upright. The pain in my head magnified unbearably as I collapsed onto the floor. I though of calling out to Lourdes, whose kitchen window was just a few feet from the side of the house (she and Lydia often carried on animated conversations from their respective houses). But still, I couldn't muster the strength. *And besides*, I thought in a tiny moment of clarity, *she'll just panic and insist on hauling me off to the hospital and all I really want right now is to go back to bed and not move anymore.* After a few minutes, I fought to pull myself up and staggered back to bed. I would go see the doctor in the morning.

The Family Doctor

I awoke early the next morning, roused from sleep by the sharp squeals of the neighbor's pig. Foggily, I recalled the events of the previous night, and was relieved to discover my head had returned to its normal state, had not exploded during the night, and was, in fact, still securely attached to my neck. I swung my legs out of bed and stood up on the cool tile floor. An immediate jolt of pain shot through my feet. The bones, I realized, felt painfully inflamed.

I forced myself to eat a small breakfast, wincing at the loud pops in my joints as I moved about the kitchen. The sounds made me think of a line from an old Rice Krispies jingle. *It's time to put some snap, crackle, pop into your morning!* I sat in the rocking chair for the better part of the morning, idly humming this absurd line, trying to summon the courage to go see the family doctor up the street.

"Katherine!" exclaimed the doctor as I poked my head in her consulting room. "How terrible of you to go a whole week without visiting us."

I was glad to note the consulting room was empty of the usual assortment of visiting friends, neighbors, children and patients. "Actually, Melbita," I said hesitantly as I sat down, "I didn't come here today to observe. I came as a patient . . . you see, I haven't been feeling very well . . . " I trailed off.

"Oh no, what's wrong?" she asked concerned.

"Well, last week I had this terrible sore throat and fatigue. It went away for a few days, but now it's come back. And then I had this terrible headache last night. It was just awful, I thought I was going to die. And now all my bones hurt and I have a fever. I'm so tired I can hardly move . . . "

She looked immediately concerned. "Oh, Katherine," she said softly, biting her lip. "Oh, I'm so sorry you're sick."

"What do you think I have," I asked her pointedly. "Is it dengue?"

She looked at me silently for a moment. "No, no it's not dengue. There's this virus going around . . . " she trailed off.

"What should I do?" I asked her.

"Oh, Katherine, I'm so glad you came to see me in my clinic about this. You really are my friend, you know, and I wish I could take care of you as my patient, but this actually isn't the family doctor clinic that serves your house." She got up from her desk. "Come on, I'll walk you over to your family doctor's. I'm surprised you haven't met her yet, she's an old friend of mine from the university and I promise she'll take good care of you." She took me by the arm and walked with me to a nearby clinic.

"This is Katherine, she's an *American*," Melba said, peeking her head in the office of a nearby *consultorio*. A startled-looking woman in a white lab coat stared back at us. "She's living here and studying at the university," Melba continued. "Did you know you had an American living in your zone?"

"No," came the muted response. I couldn't help but notice how apprehensive this new doctor looked, as if she would rather deal with just about anything other than a sick American living in her zone.

"Katherine came to see me because she's been feeling very sick and she's a friend of mine, but I'm bringing her here because she's in YOUR zone," Melba continued. It was hard to miss the unstated meaning of this exchange. Melba turned back to me with a maternal smile. "Now Mary, I'm putting you in very good hands. Doctora Veronica and I have been friends since the university. She'll take good care of you." With an audible sigh of relief, she turned and left.

The doctor, still stunned and unsmiling, motioned for me to sit down and began asking me the usual assortment of medical history questions, then wordlessly wrote out two lab requests for blood analysis. Numbly I clutched my little slips of paper and made my way home. I had been instructed to go to the policlinic, but the thought of having blood drawn with a reusable glass syringe filled me with dread. No sense in compounding the situation by getting hepatitis or meningitis, I muttered darkly, and went to look up the number of the "International" (foreigners only) health clinic in my Cuba guidebook.

The International Clinic

The international clinic (which the guidebook had assured me was "excellent quality, open 24 hours, and has English-speaking staff") was located in a small house atop one of Santiago's most imposing hillsides. The clinic appeared quite vacant, except for a handful of employees seated on the couch in the air-conditioned lobby watching the end of a bad karate movie on HBO (the international clinic, like all facilities for foreigners, was provided with pirated American cable TV).

I had been overtaken by terrible nausea in the short car-ride, and sank silently into the soft leather couch in front of the TV and tried to keep from vomiting. A tall, statuesque doctor emerged and introduced herself, and my neighbor (who had given me a ride) was kind enough to explain my situation to her. The doctor smiled at me and explained that the blood technician had gone out for lunch so I would have to wait for a bit. Few things had ever felt better to me than that soft leather couch in the air-conditioned lobby. I could have gladly spent the whole day there.

A few moments later the movie finished, the staff dispersed and someone handed me the remote control for the TV. Curious, I flipped through the channels and found CNN. The culture shock was immediate and profound. For several months my life had been characterized by scorching sun, sweat, dirt, scarcity and the deep timelessness of Santiago. CNN was so glittery and dazzling that for a moment I could hardly imagine that it came from a real world at all. I began to understand why Cubans were always talking of "La Yuma[1]" in such hushed, awed tones. It hovered like a sparkling mirage on the horizon.

The blood technician entered, abruptly interrupting my reverie, and escorted me back to a small examination room where he calmly drew a vial of blood, analyzed it, and told me everything was fine. I didn't have dengue after all. It was probably just hepatitis.

I returned to the house and fell into a woozy sleep. A few hours later, two family doctors (my family doctor and another woman I didn't know) showed up with grim faces, and asked to see the lab report. They took it and hastily retreated to a far corner of the front porch, murmuring conspiratorially to each and pointing to several of the numbers.

The doctors deluged me with more questions—did I have fever? Headaches? Normal menstruation? Bleeding from gums? Vomiting? I lied and stubbornly insisted I didn't feel so bad. They ignored my protests and instead made me lie down on the bed so that they could poke at my liver.

Following this, they again retreated to the porch and began a long whispered conversation with each other. Curious, I tried to get close enough to eavesdrop, but they broke apart before I could hear anything. Lisette went back to the phone and made more hushed calls. I managed to make out disjointed bits of conversation— "We have a patient," "platelets are low," "liver," "foreigner" and (most frightening) "hospital."

I began to get very tense. "Just what do you think I have?" I asked pointedly to the other doctor, who was sitting in the rocking chair across from me.

She hemmed and hawed. "Well, there's this virus going around. Usually what we do is put the patient in the hospital for a few days just to observe."

"Hospital!" I squawked. "I don't want to go to any hospital. I'm not that sick." My protests again fell on deaf ears. Lisette hung up the phone and said we must wait until "they" called her back. We all sat in the rockers and stared at one another. The minutes ticked by. Finally the phone rang. Lisette muttered, nodded and hung up.

"Well?" I asked. More silence. "Do I have to go to the hospital or not?"

"Well, we're not sure since you're a foreigner. They're sending most everybody to the *clinico-quirujico* [Santiago's newest hospital]. But we may have to send you to the international clinic. They're going to call back in a few minutes." Again we sat in silence while I tried to assimilate the fact that I had no say in this matter.

"And how long are they going to keep me there?" I heard my voice getting more subdued. I was just too tired to stay angry for very long.

"Oh, not long," they said smoothly. "Five or six days."

"Five or six days!" I shouted. "But I'm not really very sick."

"Maybe even less. Maybe three for four. Don't worry, it's only for observation." They sounded slick and crafty and I didn't believe them for a minute. I sat back and tried keep from panicking.

The phone rang again. There were more hushed conversations. I managed to make out, "Hospital," foreigner" and "transport."

"So when do I have to go?" I asked, trying to plan how I was going to spend my last night in the house.

"The ambulance should be here in a little while."

"Ambulance!" I shouted. "I don't need an ambulance." I was met only with more expressionless stares. I knew in most Cuban hospitals patients had to bring their own sheets and towels, and usually a full-time companion to bring them food since the hospital food was rumored to be vile. How was I going to get word out? Phone calls from Cuba to the U.S. sometimes took as long as two hours to go through. I didn't have two hours.

The ambulance never arrived, and a neighbor was tasked with driving me to the international clinic. He left me at the door, reassuring me that his daughter lived nearby and would check on me in the evening so I wouldn't feel so alone. But still, a wave of fear washed over as I stepped out of the car, my little bundle of provisions clutched tightly in my aching hands.

A few moments later, a white jeep pulled up in front of the clinic and the doctor gestured for me to get up and follow her outside. As I tried to stand up I realized that I was unbearably exhausted. The weight of my little bag seemed to be bruising the bones in my hand as I struggled to lift it. "Where are we going?" I asked fatalistically. Perhaps they were going to whisk me away to some secret interrogation room and bludgeon me with truncheons.

"We've decided to send you on to the hospital with the other patients," the nurse said evasively. "We really only have one little consulting room here. We're just not set up for inpatients. You'll be better off at the hospital."

I tossed my little bag in the jeep, fighting panic once again, though this time my fear had been largely replaced with exhausted resignation. "Will I need any syringes or anything?" the practical part of my brain prompted me to ask.

The doctor stopped and looked at me for a second. "You mean you don't have any?" It was not so much a question as an accusation.

"No."

"Wait here," she ordered, and ran inside. A few moments later she emerged and thrust a handful of disposable syringes in my hands. "Here's five, that should be enough."

"Thanks," I muttered, gripping them numbly. The driver started the jeep with a roar and careened down a back road toward the main hospital. I felt a shudder of fear as we drove past a large, barbed-wired military post and tried to suppress mental images of horrible Dickensonian hospitals and little dank torture cells. The bumps in the road jolted my hip bones painfully against the seat.

"Is there a phone in the hospital I could use?" I ask timidly.

"I think there's probably one in the entranceway," the doctor said. "But there's none in the ward, and once you go in there you can't go out again."

Great, I thought morosely. They are sending me to jail.

Hospital

The doctor walked with me into the hospital and left me alone in the crowded admissions area—a large circle of rusty folding lawn chairs in a green-tiled room off the main entranceway. The metal frame of the chair dug painfully into my tender bones as I settled in to wait. Feverish and weak, I struggled to control my growing fear at the grim spectacle unfolding around me. The room was full of dreadfully sick people, all with dull, sunken eyes and vacant stares. One old woman lay slumped over the admissions table dead to the world. Another dozed quietly, clutching an ancient portable fan in her lap. The harsh fluorescent light reflecting off the walls cast the whole room in a sickly pallor. Moments passed. A young woman vomited into a wastebasket in the corridor. A bored-looking admissions nurse wrote mindlessly on scattered slips paper. Hungry mosquitoes buzzed around my ankles.

I looked down and contemplated my aching bones. The feel of them kept reminding of an old horror story by Ray Bradbury about a man with a terribly painful . . . well, *problem* with his skeleton. Dengue, I decided, was not unlike that. Perhaps it should rightfully be known as "skeleton's disease" instead of "breakbone fever." After all, it isn't so much the individual bones that hurt, but one's whole internal frame that feels sick and fragile and infected, as if the tiniest blow might shatter it altogether.

I jumped, startled out of my morbid reverie as the bored-looking admissions nurse finally called my name. I walked resignedly to the desk and recited all my symptoms while she scribbled everything down on the back of a piece of old computer paper without looking at me. An orderly was called to escort me to the room.

"Can I use the phone?" I asked him. I knew it would be my last chance to get any word out about my forced hospitalization.

"Oh, there isn't any phone." He yawned.

"How can a hospital this big and this modern not have a phone?" I asked reproachfully.

He paused for a moment. "I think there may be a pay phone outside." His expression indicated he didn't particularly care one way or another.

The pay phone was broken, but he led me to another on the second floor. After several tries, I managed to get a call through to one of my neighbors and asked him to call Atlanta for me and explain what was happening. It felt as desperate and hopeless as putting a note in a bottle to cross the Straits of Florida.

Following this brief excursion, I was led upstairs to dengue (or "virus") ward number five. An armed soldier guarded the door, and for a moment I was filled with an odd thrill of discovery—knowing that what I was about to see was officially nonexistent. My inner anthropologist was quite delighted—to my knowledge no foreign researcher had ever had such an experience in Cuba before. The rest of me remained sick, exhausted and afraid.

We passed first through the men's ward. A few patients clad in identical white pajamas lounged around the hall. I peeked into the rooms and saw row upon row of beds, full of feverish glassy-eyed men in various stages of undress in the sweltering heat. We passed through another set of doors into the women's ward, where everyone was clad in identical white institutional gowns. The effect was grim and prison-like.

A surly nurse looked over my admission paper and directed me to bed number three in room number five. Tentatively I walked into a large collective room and put my bag down on the floor underneath the bed. There were eight narrow beds in the room, all crammed very close together with barely enough space to walk between them. Three folding chairs were squeezed into the aisle by the windows. Mosquito nets hung clumsily from wooden stakes tied to the bedposts. I decided I would feel silly climbing into bed with my clothes on and went and sat in a folding chair instead, even though the metal frame was acutely painful on my sore bones.

I looked around the room. The *Clinico-Quirujico* was a new hospital and by Cuban standards was fairly well-appointed. The beds had sheets, the electricity was on, the fixtures were clean and modern, and there was running water. Sixteen patients shared one large bathroom that consisted of two toilet stalls, two sinks and two showers (with no soap or toilet paper). The hospital was designed to maximize ventilation, and a large row of windows looked out over a central courtyard. There was no air-conditioning or fans, though, and the air was hot and stale.

The woman in the bed next to me uttered a low groan and I looked over and noticed she was hooked up to an IV on a ancient wooden stand. "*Cojones*," she shouted for all the world to hear. "This IV hurts like a son-of-a-bitch."

"Laila, try not to move your hand like that, you're bleeding into the IV line," another patient folding a towel said gently back to her. They were the only two patients in the room who were conscious. Three others lay in bed, dead to the world.

"Screw the IV," Laila growled back.

I looked over at Laila and it was obvious that she was not faring well. She was middle-aged and fat and her face has a smudged pallid look that made me uneasy about her chances for recovery. An angry rash covered her feet and legs. She looked back at me. "Don't put your bag on the floor. You can't put anything on the floor here." I obediently get up and moved the bag to a little table between our two beds.

"I just got here," I said hesitantly. I felt awkward and out of place.

"You don't look too sick. Are you sure you're in the right place?" The blonde matronly woman came and sat in the chair beside me. She folded her white hospital gown down so that the sleeves rested under her arms and the front lay over her chest, then took an old piece of cardboard and began fanning herself. "*Ai, mi madre, que calor.*" She gave me a smile. "Hello, I'm Bianca."

"*Encantada.*" I smiled back weakly. "I'm Mary Katherine. They said they wanted to put me in for observation. Honestly, it seems a little extreme, I just feel like I have a virus or something. Maybe hepatitis. But not dengue." My denial flared stubbornly in the face of so much human misery.

"Oh, well I've sure got it," Laila moaned from her bed. "*cojones*, my legs itch like a son-of-a-bitch."

"Laila is the president of our room," Bianca laughed. "Look how sick she is and she still spends the whole day making jokes."

"*Cojones*," Laila growled, then laughed as well. I noted with some apprehension that she appeared to have no teeth.

"And I'm the vice-president," Bianca added solemnly. "Two of our ministers went home today, so we're all that's left of this administration."

"Can I be a minister too?" I ask with a smile. Already I liked these women and felt myself drawing strength from their gentle humor.

"Look, Laila, she wants to be a minister!" Bianca was clearly delighted by the idea.

"I'll have to be minister of international relations," I said thoughtfully, "Since I'm a foreigner."

Laila laughed loudly. "Hey, Maria," she hollered to a sickly looking old woman standing in the doorway, "Come meet Katherine, our new Minister of International Relations." Maria shuffled over, clutching her hospital gown at the front. She seemed a bit intimidated by the boisterous banter and silently took a seat in the last folding chair by the window.

"Where are you from?" Bianca asked me.

I smiled. "The U.S."

"An American! What are you doing here in Cuba? Vacationing?"

"No, no. I'm not a tourist. I'm a student at the University."

"Our minister of foreign relations is an American?" Laila was clearly excited by the novelty of meeting an American. "*Cojones*! What are you studying?"

"*Ciencias sociales.*"

"Ahhh. Social sciences," they all repeated to each other, nodding earnestly.

"Hey nurse," Laila bellowed at the top of her lungs. "Come and meet Katherine. She's from the United States, studying at the university in *ciencias sociales.*"

The surly nurse wandered in. "Laila, watch that mouth of yours. You need to give it a rest." Laila made a face at her. The nurse handed me a white hospital gown. "Here put this on in the bathroom," she growled.

My reaction to the gown was entirely irrational. It infuriated me and I refused to put it on. "No," I said stubbornly.

"What?" The nurse looked incredulous, as if she couldn't quite grasp the fact that I had disagreed with her.

"I'm not all that sick," I heard myself whining. "Why can't I just wear my regular clothes?" The nurse's expression informed me that she really didn't give a damn what I wore, but wasn't going to put up with any argument.

"Just put it on," she said harshly.

"Put it on," Bianca said, giving me a puzzled look. "It's just a gown."

Sensing further argument would be futile, I went grumbling into the bathroom. My skin felt flushed and hot as I slipped off my dress. The gown was made of thick cotton and reminded me of the heavy sheets my grandmother used in the winter. I felt distinctly unglamorous, but since there was no mirror in the bathroom I couldn't honestly appraise myself. I slowly shuffled out, grateful that (unlike American hospital gowns) there were no embarrassing gaps in the back. Laila and Bianca applauded. To amuse them I struck a Vogue pose. They whistled and hollered. "Latest fashion," I said ruefully, taking my seat again.

Putting on the gown affected me profoundly. Bit by bit, minute by minute I felt my entire sense of self slipping away—felt myself being consumed by the institution and my new singular identity as a patient. From that moment on I really felt like nobody at all—just another invisible figure, held incommunicado with a politically incorrect case of "virus."

My body reacted remarkably to the hospital gown as well. As I sat and looked down, listening to Laila and Bianca's feisty banter flow around me, the pain in my bones seemed to grow unbearable, my gaze more spacy and feverish, my fatigue overwhelming. My body, whose symptoms had been denied for so long, appeared to view the donning of the gown as definitive permission to become officially sick. I tottered over to the bed and lay down, overcome with misery.

* * *

"*Cojones*," shouted Laila a short while later, waking me out of a fitful doze. "These mosquito nets are *de carajo*. Too hot." She began fanning herself with an old piece of cardboard.

"Why do they have mosquito nets?" I asked sleepily.

"So the mosquitoes won't bite us," Laila said with a straight face. I looked around the room. Everyone had cast their nets off because of the heat, and mosquitoes were everywhere.

"Oh, Katherine, you should have been here yesterday when we had the *despedida* (going-away party) for our other two ministers," Bianca said gaily. "One of them took her mosquito net and wound it all around her head, so it trailed down her back, like a bridal train. Then she took another and wrapped it around her shoulders. We all did her makeup and I braided her hair up on top of her head. She did herself up so beautifully! Just like a bride. We sent her off down the hallway and sang the Wedding song. The women in the cafeteria even threw some rice at her. Everybody in the whole ward came and paid tribute, and we all shared our cookies and had a real party. It was a wonderful diversion."

I smiled in awe at the magical nature of Cubans—the only people in the world festive enough to transform a plague ward into a slumber party.

"Katherine, how do you say *cojones* in English?" Laila asked me suddenly.

"Balls," I said, grateful for the way they were diverting my attention.

"How is it?" she asked eagerly. "Boolss?"

"No, Ballz." I said emphasizing the Z sound at the end.

"Ah, Bahlss." She appeared quite pleased with this addition to her vocabulary and practiced it diligently, always exaggerating the s sound on the end.

"I only know how to say one thing in English," Bianca volunteered primly, still fanning herself in the folding chair. "That's 'yes'."

"Ah, look at what a whore she is," Laila cracked, "all she can say is yes."

I laughed. "'No' is the same in English as in Spanish. Now you can say both yes and no."

"Yes," Bianca said solemnly.

"No," I answered pointedly.

"Bahllss," shouted Laila.

A young nurse's aid with rotting teeth walked by the room and shouted "*Merienda*." I stayed in bed, unsure of what to do.

"Hey," Laila shouted at her, "Come and meet Katherine." The girl poked her head back into the room. "She's from the United States and she's here studying in *ciencias sociales*," Laila explained.

"*Mucho gusto*," the girl said shyly, backing nervously out the door-way. I guessed she was another one who had never actually seen an American before.

"My specialty in the university was philosophy," Maria, the old woman by the window, suddenly piped up. I was surprised to hear her speak.

"I don't have a specialty," Laila scowled.

"Oh, yes you do," I laughed, a wicked pun forming in my head.

"Really? What?" she demanded.

"Laila, you're an expert in . . . Ciencias *Cojonales*," I said, laughing hard at my own joke. Everyone in the room was convulsed with laugh-ter for several minutes. It was some time before Laila was even able to speak. Laughing felt good. I felt momentarily human again.

"Come, let's go and get our snack," Bianca said when all the excite-ment had died down.

"Yes, I've hardly eaten all day." I was hungry, although the thought of getting out of bed seemed difficult if not impossible.

"Get your glass and let's go. Laila, I'm going to bring you your snack now."

"I don't have a glass," I said, wishing somebody had told me a little more carefully what I needed to bring.

"They didn't tell you to bring a glass? Did you bring a spoon?"

"No. Nobody told me anything."

Bianca shook her head and remained silent—a typical Cuban response to the impulse to criticize people in authority. She asked around until she found a glass and a spoon for me to borrow.

In order to be fed, all the patients had to get up and walk to the cafeteria at the end of the ward. Those too sick to move had to depend on other patients to bring them food or be left without. There appeared to be only one nurse for the entire ward, and she rarely stirred from the nurse's station.

"Don't be afraid to yell if something hurts," Bianca counseled me as we walked to the cafeteria. "You have to yell to get their attention, otherwise they'll ignore you. Yell loudly, like this—'it hurts here,' or 'I'm bleeding here.'"

I winced at the thought of having to yell for nursing care and silently prayed my condition wouldn't worsen. I knew it was possible to develop potentially fatal complications from even a mild case of dengue—a serious hemorrhage could occur instantly and without warning. I shuddered at the thought of what might happen if I took a turn for the worse. Given that the epidemic officially didn't exist I had no doubt that the Cubans would resist informing anyone about my whereabouts or my condition. Most likely, I brooded darkly, they would just send my body back home with some tire marks on it and tell my parents how sorry they were that I had been run over by a truck.

"Are there any doctors here?" I asked Bianca.

"Oh, sure. I think there's one anyway," she said absently as we took our place in the cafeteria line. "They'll probably come and pester you tomorrow."

Bianca took Laila her glass of cereal and a cookie and set them on the little bedside table we shared. "Don't you want your cereal, Laila?" she asked.

"*Cojones,* I'm sick of cereal," Laila muttered. "Help me to the bathroom."

Bianca immediately put down her glass and went over to Laila's bed, gently unhooking the IV from the wooden stand (which had no wheels) and held it behind Laila's lumbering form while they gingerly made their way to the bathroom. "Don't lower your arm," Bianca reprimanded. "You're bleeding into the line." I could see the IV line had filled up with blood, and realized Laila's platelet count must be dangerously low.

"*Cojones,*" Laila muttered. Bianca followed along beside her, holding the IV over her head and making light conversation to distract Laila from her pain and discomfort. As they made their way gingerly to the bathroom I noticed a constellation of ugly red smudges on the back of Laila's white hospital gown and realized with some revulsion that she was hemorrhaging through her skin.

"Did you have a lot of bleeding?" I asked Bianca nervously after they returned from the bathroom.

"No, not really," she said. "But I sure had all the other symptoms. Oh, when I got here to the hospital I could hardly walk. I couldn't see and I was vomiting all the time. It was terrible. I still have a lot of pain in my legs, but I should be going home tomorrow," she sighed hopefully. "I've already been here almost a week. They don't let you go home until your fever goes away and your platelets are normal. I barely had any fever at all yesterday."

I immediately gobbled down two Advil to try and reduce my fever, hoping I could fake my way into an early release.

"I've been here a week already," Laila grouched. "And I'm not getting any better. I have bad complications with my lungs, and all this bleeding . . . And after three days with this damned IV, all the fluid's making me bloat up like a pig. *Ai, cojones esa picasón!*" she swore, scratching at her inflamed legs with her cardboard.

"Is that normal, the rash and itching?" I asked. Since it didn't look like I would be seeing a doctor anytime soon, I was eager to learn about my prognosis from the other patients.

"Well," Bianca mused, "I think seven to ten days of being sick is normal. First you get the aches and fever, then the rash. Not everybody gets the bleeding, sometimes your platelet count just drops a little. Do you have any red spots?" she asked me.

"I don't know," I replied. "The doctors kept poking at my arms and looking for something, but they didn't tell me anything. They just said it was a virus."

Laila gave a loud snort. "*Cojones*," she muttered. "A virus."

"Here, let me see,' Bianca said, walking over to my bed. She took my arm and inspected it carefully. "Hmmmm." She turned it over to look at the soft white skin underneath. "That looks like a spot, and there," she said, poking at a couple of suspicious looking red spots. "Do you have fever?" she asked. "Aches and pains?"

"Yes, lots of aches and a low fever. Actually, I was sick last week, but it went away. Then it came back last night with this terrible headache."

"We'll it sounds like you've got it all right," Bianca said firmly. "Even though you don't seem as sick as everybody else."

"It just hasn't gotten her yet," Laila smirked from the next bed.

I shuddered inwardly at the thought of growing ever sicker and more helpless with no one to take care of me. "Maybe I just have hepatitis or something," I ventured. "If it's dengue why haven't they publicized it, to warn people?"

Both Bianca and Laila remained uneasily silent, and I realized that I had strayed into politically sensitive terrain. No matter what they might think privately, no one could afford to be overheard criticizing the government in front of an American.

One of the sleeping patients had woken up and blinked owlishly as she handed the nurse her thermometer. She had ugly black smudges under her eyes and looked painfully dehydrated. "Your temperature's forty degrees [102]," the nurse scowled at her as she looked at the thermometer. "Go get some ice, soak a towel in it and wrap it around your neck."

"*Ai, Dios mio*," she moaned, trying to get out of bed. "*Cuanto me duele.*" She tottered slowly down to the kitchen to ask for ice.

"Can't she take aspirin to lower her fever?" I asked.

"Oh, no," Bianca reprimanded me. "Aspirin can give you hemorrhages. There's only one kind of painkiller you can take for dengue, and I think they're almost out. With so many people sick they just don't have enough . . . " she trailed off.

I digested this unsettling bit of news with some trepidation. If I had taken aspirin for my headache the night before I could very well have developed a fatal hemorrhage. Again the stupidity of failing to publicize this epidemic and the potentially fatal complications that were likely to result from the overall negligence infuriated me. Aspirin was the only readily available pain reliever in Cuba these days. How many people might die simply because the government refused to acknowledge this increasingly serious epidemic for the sake of its own boasting about having eradicated dengue? And what about the tourists? If they weren't telling the Cubans about it, then surely they wouldn't warn the tourists either. A major trade fair, the ExpoCaribe was scheduled for mid-June and thousands of foreign visitors were expected. How many of them would needlessly fall sick (or worse, unknowingly take the virus home with them) because they weren't warned to take precautions?

I lay in my bed, staring up at the white mosquito net, brooding nervously about the terrible situation I had fallen into. Two mosquitoes trapped in a corner of the net looked back at me. Laila, whose bed was next to the window, was besieged by hordes of mosquitoes that feasted on the pinprick hemorrhages on her legs, making her moan miserably throughout the evening.

A persistent fantasy kept replaying itself in my mind as I drifted in and out of consciousness: a kind, benevolent doctor (whom I imagined looking like a cross between Cary Grant and Ricardo Montalban) would suddenly appear at my bedside and endeavor to explain everything about dengue (its course, prognosis, and outcome) in beautiful fluent English. He would pat my hand and say, "don't worry, you'll be fine." Tomorrow, I kept thinking, surely they'll let me talk to a doctor who will explain things to me.

Laila's loud cries woke me abruptly once again. I looked over and saw Bianca tending to her legs. "*Cojones*, get these damned mosquitoes off me," she wailed, waving the frayed piece of cardboard. I looked at my watch. It was only 10:30 P.M.

"Daisy, try not to move your arm like that, you're bleeding into the IV line again," Bianca said gently.

I closed my eyes tightly and tried not to listen. I simply didn't think I could cope with any more blood or fear or agony.

"You know, Laila," Bianca said encouragingly, "Tomorrow they might move you to a special room. You know, where they'll bring you all your meals and you'll have your very own nurse to look after you."

I had a bad feeling about what this might mean for Laila's chances of survival. No doubt the critical patients were moved to a separate ward before they died. Her physical appearance was so poor, and she seemed to have so many complications that I figured her chances weren't good.

"*Ai, tengo sangramiento*, ("I have bleeding") Laila moaned, clasping her belly.

"Come on, we'll go into the bathroom," Bianca said, unhooking her IV bottle from the stand and helping her out of bed.

"Can I help?" I finally asked. I was one of the more ambulatory patients in the ward and was starting to feel guilty just lying in bed pretending to sleep.

"Could you go ask the nurse for some cotton?" Bianca called back over her shoulder as they gingerly made their way to the bathroom. I could see a small red stain, like the petal of a rose, emerging on the lower part of Laila's gown.

Another surly nurse had replaced the one who was on duty when I arrived. She sat behind a tall counter in the center of the ward and regarded me with no small amount of annoyance as I approached her. "Could I have some cotton?" I asked meekly.

"Are you bleeding?" she said.

"No, it's for Laila."

Wordlessly she reached into a drawer and handed me a packet of sterile cotton.

I returned to the room and saw Laila was back in bed. I looked in the bathroom and saw Bianca washing out Laila's abundant bloomers in the sink. I couldn't help but notice the trash can by the toilet was overflowing with dark, bloody lengths of cotton. "The nurse gave me this," I said weakly, waving the packet.

"Thanks, Mary," Laila muttered. "*Cojones, que pena.*"

I found myself strangely awake after this incident. I felt nervous and restless and took to pacing up and down the hall, hoping to calm myself down. The nurses had turned out the lights in the rooms, leaving only one weak incandescent bulb burning in the hallway. Up and down I went in the dim light. After about the third pass, the nurse began to get irked with me. "What do you think you're doing?" she barked.

"I'm just restless," I replied. Actually, the more I walked, the more I realized that pacing gave me an opportunity both to calm down and to collect some useful information on the epidemic. As I walked by the rooms, I began trying to keep track of how many patients were in the ward. By the fourth pass I had counted a total of fifty beds, about thirty-nine of which were occupied. I stopped at the nurses station to ask for some water and saw a handwritten list of phone numbers for other wings that had been converted into dengue wards. I quickly counted them.

There was a total of ten wards, and assuming they all had approximately the same rate of occupancy I estimated that the hospital was currently holding around 400 dengue patients. I knew patients were also being sent to the provincial hospital and the military hospital, so there could easily be as many as 1,500 hospitalized dengue patients at that particular moment. And presumably not all sick people would be hospitalized. Given that it was a mosquito-borne disease, it would seem logical to expect the epidemic to progress exponentially.

The room was dark and quiet, but still it was many hours before I was able to fall asleep. I tossed and turned, obsessively cataloging all the bad things that might befall me if I took a turn for the worse. Again and again in the dark of night I would wake to hear plaintive cries of, "*tengo sangramiento*," up and down the ward. Often I heard Bianca's soothing voice, helping Laila to the bathroom, washing out her bloomers or just fanning some of the pestiferous mosquitoes away. The feverish girl woke twice, cried for help and then vomited loudly onto the floor. The room was often flooded with bright fluorescent light as the nurse reluctantly came to investigate some disturbance or another. I realized with profound clarity how the invention of the nurse call button completely transformed the nature of the modern hospital. All around me echoed a medieval cacophony of moans and cries.

At one point early in the morning I awoke to a wild breeze whipping through the ward. My mosquito netting blew off its stakes and settled over me like a shroud. Groggily I got up to refasten it and heard the sound of distant thunder. A rainstorm was blowing up, and I could feel a cool mist of air blowing in through the window. Santiago had been going through a terribly hot and dry summer, and the thought of a rain shower was heavenly. I lay back in bed, lulled immediately to sleep by the cool wind and the soft, gentle sound of the pouring rain.

Day Two and Beyond

My memories of subsequent days in the hospital are vague. Exhausted and in considerable pain, I kept taking codeine pills and spent much of the time in a hazy narcotics stupor unable to take any more notes. I remember being prodded awake on numerous occasions by pesky doctors and epidemiologists who interrogated me about my symptoms, my brief remission of the previous week, my travels around the city, and the number of mosquitoes I encountered in various places. None of them, however, ever once uttered the word "dengue" or answered any questions about my condition or prognosis.

Bianca, much to my and Laila's dismay, was discharged the day after I arrived. I was amused to see that she spent over an hour hunched secretively over a tiny pocket mirror putting on makeup and arranging her hair before she left.

"Look at the kind of woman she is," Laila teased her mercilessly. "You know why she's going through all that trouble, don't you?"

"No, why?" I asked mystified. Even though she was being discharged Bianca was still far from well, and I was curious as to why she was making herself up so intently just to go home and recuperate.

"She didn't tell you?" Laila guffawed. "Her boyfriend is waiting for her. And he's only eighteen years old! Look at her, *la vieja*, trying to make herself all pretty and young for him."

"Laila, you're exaggerating. He's not eighteen, he's twenty-five," Bianca said exasperatedly.

"Is that true, Bianca?" I asked her with a sly wink.

"You don't think there's anything wrong with seeing a younger man, do you Mary? I mean, he is almost twelve years younger than me." She appealed to me to arbitrate, as if my status as a foreigner gave me more authority to decide such things.

"I think it's great," I said encouragingly. "Just pace yourself, you're still not well."

"I'm well enough," she retorted.

Laila laughed loudly, then got a solemn look on her face. "But now who's going to take care of me now if you're going," she said petulantly.

"Now Laila, don't be like that. Katherine will take care of you."

"Katherine! She doesn't do anything," she pouted. I looked at her with surprise. I thought I had been doing a lot—helping her to the bathroom, fetching her cotton, washing out her glass and spoon. I had even loaned her my portable cassette player, which she stubbornly refused to return. But apparently my caregiving abilities still suffered in comparison to Bianca's.

"Don't worry, Laila, you'll be fine. I think they're even going to take you off the IV tonight." With that Bianca gathered her things, wished everybody health, and went on her way.

Bianca's departure threw the entire room into a glum mood. Three new patients had been admitted, all too sick to move or talk. Without Bianca there was no way to sustain the usual lighthearted banter that had kept us all from falling into depressed silence.

"Well, don't just lie there, " I griped to Laila, wanting some of her typical comic relief. "Talk to me. Tell me something."

"Oh, Katherine, I'm so afraid I'm going to die. I'm so sick." I wasn't prepared for this sudden seriousness. "My daughter's already twenty-one," Laila continued fitfully, "she's grown, but I have two little grandchildren who still need me to look after them. *Coño*, I've been here a week and everything still hurts—my head, my arms, my hands. When I got here I couldn't even see, couldn't walk, couldn't keep any food down. Oh, *Dios*, what a nightmare . . . I'm so afraid for my little grandsons, with no one to look after them . . . "

I looked at her and had no idea what to say. She looked so deathly ill, lying there in her hospital bed. Her skin was white and pallid, and with ugly smudges under her eyes, and tiny blossoms of blood speckled across her hospital gown. Her legs and feet were swollen and red. I groped desperately for a response, but could think of nothing at all to say.

Release

I was finally released from the hospital after three days. As usual, the reasons for my early release were never explained, and I could only assume that my fever-hiding ploy had been successful. In any event, I was ecstatic at the prospect of freedom, and hastily gathered my things, said a hurried good-bye to the other patients and the surly nurses, gave away the remainder of my Advil and codeine pills to Laila, and went to wait by the nurses station for the orderly to accompany me downstairs.

The excitement, unfortunately, was premature. I waited by the nurses station for two hours, but no one showed up to escort me out, and I was not allowed to pass the officer guarding the door unaccompanied. Wearily, I returned to the room and crawled back into bed, depressed at the thought of having to spend another night in the hospital after all.

Some time later I was awakened by Laila's gleeful cheering. They had taken her off the IV the previous day, and she took great delight in her newfound ability to move freely about the ward. "Katherine," she exclaimed, poking me in the ribs. "I'm going home too!"

"What? Today?" I gasped with surprise, but she was already dancing over to the other patients' beds, sharing her excitement. I couldn't believe they would send her home already. She had improved markedly since they took her off the IV, and had stopped hemorrhaging, but was still pale and weak. We both gathered our things and went to sit by the nurses station. I marveled at how different it felt to be in my own clothes again. Laila seemed a different person as well—stronger and more alive.

After another hour, a tired, overworked doctor finally showed up with our discharge papers. He walked us down to the same green tiled room where I was first admitted, and (after inviting me to come visit him in his clinic) turned me over to another overworked bureaucrat who spent an hour preparing a work exemption form for me. I kept trying to tell her I didn't have a formal job in Cuba, but she didn't seem to hear. As soon as the form had all the appropriate stamps on it, she curtly informed me that I was allotted seven days of rest, and after that must report back to work. I surmised that she had simply never met a foreigner before, and couldn't quite grasp the concept of anyone being exempt from the state's confining labor laws.

Laila and I were both discharged at the same time, and her family arrived and swarmed around her. She took great pride in introducing me as the foreigner who had kept her company, given her miraculous codeine pills, and made funny jokes. Her family outdid themselves in thanking me, and insisted that they be allowed to give me a ride home in their car.

As we all piled haphazardly into an ancient DeSoto, I looked curiously over the discharge papers in my hand. "What does that say?" I asked Laila's sister, unable to make out the handwriting under the "diagnosis" section.

"It says, 'virus.' You know, the '*virus*,'" she said with an exaggerated wink.

"A toast to Laila's good health!" shouted Laila's corpulent brother, who was driving wildly through the back streets of Santiago while trying to uncap a bottle of rum with his teeth.

"Ah, you brought rum," Laila squealed with delight, seizing the bottle and opening it herself. "Katherine, have some rum to celebrate with me," she made an elaborate toast and shoved the bottle in my hands. It seemed futile to suggest that maybe strong drink was not medically advisable under the circumstances. I toasted everyone's health and tipped the bottle up to my lips for a long burning draught. It was heavenly. It tasted of freedom.

The Underground Epidemic

The rain that began my first night in the hospital grew into a torrential tropical depression that lingered over Santiago for many days, flooding roads and washing away many of the flimsy shanties that covered the hillsides around the city. Water filled the streets, pooled in stagnant gray lakes. Military trucks passed through like partially submerged submarines, their headlights casting eerie green reflections from under the eddies. Few people ventured outdoors. I escaped into a tattered copy of *The Mayor of Castorbridge* I had found in a bookstore several months previously and hardly stirred from my room except to eat or watch the afternoon matinee on television. Although my fever was gone, I still suffered considerable aches and pains and was too weak even to walk next door and return soup pots.

Despite my ongoing weakness and fatigue, the constant stream of visitors through the house (including doctors I had been working with, all of whom had been very worried about me) kept me abreast of what was happening with the epidemic. About two weeks after my hospitalization one doctor informed me that the epidemic had gotten so out of control that all of the hospitals in Santiago were full beyond capacity, and cots were being set up in the neighborhood clinics to hold the overflow. Extra rations were being delivered to the state stores in anticipation of a general quarantine. Cases of dengue were rumored to be showing up in Cobre, Palma Soriano, El Caney and other outlying towns.

On June 12, rumors began circulating that unless there was a drastic drop in cases by the end of the week, the whole city would be placed under quarantine for thirty days. All events and conferences would be temporarily suspended, and (the most dramatic news of all), Fidel himself was coming to personally supervise the dengue eradication efforts.

Once mobilized, the public health effort was quite impressive. Together with a cadre of nurses, the CDR began intensively canvassing the neighborhood for anyone with signs of dengue (although they were still not allowed to identify it as such) and to eradicate domestic waste that might facilitate mosquito propagation. Planes flew overhead all day, trailing plumes of insecticide. New chemicals were imported from Canada, and men with high-tech motorized sprayers appeared at the door three times in one week to fumigate the house and patio. Civil defense tunnels were identified as a major mosquito breeding ground and were targeted for intensive spraying as well.

As the tremendous scope of the epidemic became increasingly apparent, many people in the neighborhood became irritated at being forced to maintain the charade of secrecy and denial. One neighbor visited and excitedly reported that she heard a doctor had actually begun telling his patients they had dengue, and had subsequently been censured by his superiors. "Can you imagine?" she said angrily, throwing her hands in the air. "I don't know why they don't tell us what's really going on. You know what I heard Fulano's brother say the other day? He's a bigwig in the Party and he actually tried to defend this secrecy! He said, 'We have to hide the epidemic. Otherwise it'll hurt the tourism.' Can you imagine the stupidity! If even one tourist gets sick from this, or one businessmen at the ExpoCaribe then there's going to be hell to pay." She stopped abruptly. "Of course I didn't say anything to him," she said, rolling her eyes, "or . . . you know," With a forced laugh, she pantomimed a pair of handcuff encircling her wrists.

Melba, the family doctor I had first gone to see when I began feeling sick, also stopped by and apologized profusely for not telling me I had dengue. "Oh, Katherine," she sighed sadly, "when you asked me what it was that you had, I felt so bad, but I couldn't tell you. What could I say? At first, you know, they were predicting that thousands of people in Santiago were going to die. Thankfully it's gotten somewhat stabilized now, but still . . . "

As upset as I had been at the time, there was still no way I could hold a grudge against her. I knew the penalties she was likely to face for revealing such a potentially explosive secret to an American. At the very least she would have lost her job. "I know you couldn't tell me," I reassured her. "I think it's wrong to keep an epidemic like this a secret, but I know there's nothing you can do about it."

She seemed relieved that I wasn't angry and went on, perhaps out of guilt, to pass on the latest news she had received about the course of the epidemic. "The last report I got said there's only been eight deaths, but all the doctors are saying it has to be much higher. People are scared," she said, shaking her head. "They aren't used to being sick like this."

The Official Epidemic

It wasn't until ten days after my discharge from the hospital that the local newspaper (*Sierra Maestra*) finally hinted that there might be a problem with mosquitoes in Santiago. Instead of mentioning dengue though, it stated euphemistically that "positive cases of *Aedes aegypti*" [not dengue itself, but the mosquito that causes dengue] had been detected in the neighboring towns of Palma Soriano, San Luis, Contramaestre, Songo-la Maya, Guamá and Santiago" (*Sierra Maestra*, June 14, 1997). The article went on to describe how the Aedes mosquito was capable of transmitting both dengue and yellow fever. A short description of dengue symptoms was included, along with advice on how to eliminate the mosquito from the domestic environment.

This article also reported that a battalion of over 12,000 local CDR members had been mobilized to combat the mosquito throughout the city. This brigade was responsible for policing every house to forcibly eliminate possible breeding sites such as domestic refuse or open rainwater barrels (*Sierra Maestra*, June 14, 1997). CDR members aggressively canvassed their neighborhoods, policing trash disposal and insisting that residents clean up any open bottles or patio waste that could potentially trap rainwater and harbor mosquitoes. Noncompliance was not permitted.

This extreme, militarized response was characteristic of how Cuba dealt with the devastating dengue epidemic in 1981 but with one crucial difference. At that time, a similar "health army" (*ejército de la salud*) of over 13,000 men and women had been created, and this organization, together with the regular army essentially put the country under martial law with regard to mosquito eradication (Feinsilver, 1993). In 1981, however, health education via newspapers and television had played a major role in prevention efforts. News reports of the epidemic, the eradication effort and public health advice were broadcast frequently through newspaper, radio and television. According to Feinsilver (1993),

> Particularly noteworthy was the excellent news coverage of the 1981 dengue hemorrhagic fever epidemic. . . . *Granma* ran daily articles and news items on the nature of the problem, its source, methods of eradicating the disease, and progress in stemming the epidemic and curing those already afflicted. . . . The government's ability to communicate rapidly and repeatedly with its citizens played a major role in eradicating dengue . . .

Unfortunately, this was not the case in Santiago in 1997. The city was very definitely placed under martial law with regard to mosquito eradication but there was little or no news coverage of the epidemic itself. There had not even been a public announcement that an epidemic was underway. All information on the course of the epidemic was still spread informally, through unofficial conversations or neighborhood gossip.

It wasn't until the third week of June that the local newspaper finally mentioned that there was an outbreak of dengue in Santiago, but few details were provided. The first article that appeared in *Sierra Maestra* (June 21, 1997) that mentioned the stated "*disminuye . . . el número de casos con manifestaciones de dengue y los hosptializados*" ("the number of cases and hospitalizations with signs of dengue is diminishing"). No figures were given on the number of cases reported, or the rate of new infections, although a comprehensive description of the various stages of dengue infection was provided.

Shortly after the first newspaper article on dengue was published in Santiago, the scheduled trade fair, ExpoCaribe, was held. There were some informal reports that the turnout was not as high as expected due to the news of the epidemic, but the exhibition center still appeared crowded with foreign businessmen, trade representatives and hopeful, elegantly dressed *jiniteras*. One day I walked through the ExpoCaribe and, posing as a nervous foreign girl, randomly asked a couple of visiting businessmen if they had heard anything about a dengue outbreak in Santiago. They assured me they had been told it was only a small outbreak that was already well under control.

I also approached a group of French-Canadian tourists in the lobby of the Hotel Santiago and tried the same ploy.

"Dengue?" they asked, looking puzzled. "What's that?"

"Did your tour guide say anything about taking precautions against mosquitoes?" I said, suddenly nervous that someone on the hotel staff might recognize me or overhear the conversation.

"No," they said. "Why?"

It stunned me to realize I was afraid to tell them. I didn't think they would believe me. Or else they would demand an explanation from their tour guide, who would surely insist on knowing who had been whispering such counterrevolutionary propaganda to hurt the tourism industry. If it were discovered that an American student at the University had been spreading such lies, I had no doubt things would begin to go very badly for me for the remainder of my stay. "Um . . . , " I mumbled lamely, "If you have any mosquito repellent it might be a good idea to use it." I quickly backed away and fled to the safety of the streets.

I couldn't believe what had become of me—I had become so acculturated, so effectively Cubanized, that *I* was now scared to be seen talking to foreigners! They all seemed naive and distant in their five-star hotels, air-conditioned buses and smug ignorance. I paused for a moment in dismay, suddenly aware that I had begun thinking in terms of "us" (Cubans) and "them" (tourists). But wasn't I a foreigner too? Who was "us"? Who was "them"? The gap between the two worlds I was trying to bridge seemed impossibly huge.

It didn't help my sense of disorientation that the *jiniteros* lurking outside the Hotel Santiago (thinking I was a foreigner in town for the ExpoCaribe) immediately began accosting me, trying to hustle me with the same predictable tales of helplessness and despair that inevitably softened the hearts and opened the wallets of gullible tourists. They swarmed around me like an aggressively friendly school of pirañas, offering discounted prices on cigars and rum, guide services and automobile rental in addition to constant sexual innuendo, and humble pleas for money to buy medicine for nonexistent relatives.

"I'm not a tourist," I snapped at them, desperately struggling to figure out what exactly I *was* in this sharply bifurcated world.

In the meantime, I continued to try and collect as much information as possible on the epidemic, and was pleased (though also frightened) at the way my newfound complicity encouraged people to speak openly with me. Several days after one particularly optimistic newspaper article appeared, I went to visit another doctor I knew to ask for the latest underground information. He was privately quite enraged at the way the public health authorities were handling the epidemic,

> It makes me furious that they tell these lies. Like in the paper when they say they're letting people out of the hospital at a rate of 600 per day. Well they said that three days ago, and if it were really the case the hospitals would be empty by now and they're still plenty full. All the cardiac wards, the maternity wards, everything is being converted into use for the epidemic. Plus a little while ago they asked PAHO for help [in controlling the epidemic]. Well, PAHO told them that if they're going to help they [the Cuban government] have to officially declare it's an epidemic and report how many deaths. They [the Cuban government] said they'd only had six deaths—really there's been more than fifteen—and PAHO said, "it doesn't sound like much of an epidemic to me." And now there's been another twelve cases officially diagnosed in *Havana*. Who knows what's going to happen if it takes hold there too. . . . And now they're saying "if there's no fever it's not dengue," which isn't true. There's been a bunch of cases

where people had all the symptoms, but their fever never rose above 37 [Celsius, or 99 Fahrenheit]. I guess they just want to try and make it out like there's fewer cases than there actually are.

Other doctors reiterated these sentiments, and nearly always expressed anger and frustration at the secrecy and denial that had so far characterized the epidemic. The delayed public health response, and the lack of a clear health education program seemed to be the most frequent causes of complaint. One doctor stated, "In May they were saying by June 1 it [the epidemic] would all be under control, but instead the numbers [of new cases] increased. Now they're saying it's going down, but who really knows? Supposedly they asked PAHO [the Pan American Health Organization] for help, but PAHO said they had to make an official declaration of the number of cases. They told PAHO it was only 800, but really it's more like 8,000."

It wasn't until the following week (almost a month after my hospitalization) that *Sierra Maestra* (June 28, 1997) finally featured a comprehensive article on the dengue epidemic. It reported that the number of cases had diminished remarkably, and that the public health initiative had succeeded in containing the outbreak entirely to the municipality of Santiago. Shortly after my hospitalization, in fact, (when all the doctors I knew were claiming the epidemic was still quite out of control), the national minister of public health, Carlos Dotres, claimed the outbreak of dengue had been controlled and subsequently lauded the public health measures as a great success,

We can demonstrate in Cuba and to the world that we are capable with respect to the *Aedes aegypti* and the outbreak of dengue to control, limit, and eradicate—something very difficult and seldom seen in other parts of the world . . . (*Sierra Maestra*, June 21, 1997).

Furthermore, in keeping with this official line, hospitalized patients interviewed in the local Santiago newspaper spoke glowing of the medical treatment they received, "The medical care is marvelous," one patient reported, "The doctors and nurses here with me are very concerned . . . [and] we patients feel very supported with the treatment they give us" (*Sierra Maestra*, June 21, 1997).

Note

1. "La Yuma" is a common colloquial term for the United States. It is rich in symbolic meanings, and is typically invoked to represent material abundance and technological wonders (such as computers, cellular telephones, IPods, cable television and fast food restaurants) that are conspicuously absent in Cuba. When referring to the negative aspects of the United States, Cubans typically speak of "*El Imperialismo*" rather than *La Yuma*. *La Yuma* is a place of great awe and fascination. *El Imperialismo* is dark and violent, intent on destroying Cuba with it's aggressive *bloqueo* (or trade embargo).

4

Fearful Interlude

After several weeks I had recuperated enough to resume some of my research activities, but the illness took a tremendous toll on me physically and emotionally. Whereas before I had felt quite secure in my place in the world, after the hospitalization I did not. The dengue fever epidemic was a powerful lesson in how readily the Cuban government could erase any event (or individual) that might prove politically embarrassing. It was unsettling to realize that my knowledge of this secret epidemic might put me in such a category. Would I be allowed to leave Cuba? Would they take my books, notes and computer away from me? The sudden appearance of Cuban state security personnel at my doorstep did not do much to ease my fears.

They first materialized in a little white Lada, claiming to be representatives of the "Juventude" (the Union of Young Communists—the Party's youth organization), but their aggressively friendly smiles and terrifyingly blank eyes gave them away. For some odd reason they reminded me of a Pentecostal duo named Brother Bob and Sister Cindy who used to preach on street corners in my home town in Kentucky. Watching them walk towards me, knowing that they had *come for me*, was far from reassuring. Despite these misgivings I still managed to sit impassively in my rocking chair and cordially exchange greetings.

After introducing themselves, they abruptly invited me to accompany them for the afternoon for purposes of enjoying some "cultural interchange." It was not an invitation I felt I could refuse—it seemed such an innocuous request, after all. And besides, I thought naively, I had nothing to fear—I had no contacts with any "enemies of the revolution," and no connection with the United States government—even my research funding was from private foundations. So why risk seeming hostile or uncooperative?

I said good-bye to Lydia and walked compliantly over to the little white Lada. The man (who I immediately began thinking of as Brother Bob) got behind the driver's seat and started the car, and the woman (who correspondingly became Sister Cindy) sat in the back seat with me. She was cool and unsmiling and emanated an aura of veiled hostility and contempt, reinforcing my subconscious fear that I was being taken into custody rather than being escorted to a friendly *"intercambio cultural."* I did my best to remain calm and composed, but at a certain level couldn't help but wonder if I would ever return.

Brother Bob drove to a renovated old mansion in a Santiago suburb with a "Union of Young Communists" banner prominently displayed across the front. I was led up two flights of stairs, to a small curtained room with a table in the middle. Brother Bob, still smiling his rather predatory smile, sat across from me and opened a hard bound notebook while Sister Cindy disappeared into another room, then returned a few moments later bearing two glasses of bright orange liquid.

"Here, have some *refresco,*" she muttered, placing the glasses on the table and quickly disappearing again. *Refresco* was the local equivalent of Kool-Aid—a rather sickeningly sweet concoction of sugar and artificial flavor. I looked at it and felt an irrational surge of fear. On the surface, of course, everything appeared quite innocuous, and Brother Bob and Sister Cindy appeared to be doing their best to appear hospitable and non-threatening (though with decidedly mixed success). But still, my internal alarm bells were ringing, especially at the thought of ingesting any mixture of water and powdered drink mix that these two unnervingly blank-eyed individuals put before me.

The substance of the interview, however, proved to be somewhat anticlimactic. Brother Bob wanted to know everything about how I happened to come to Cuba. Who did I know in Atlanta? Who were my contacts in Havana? Who had sent me? What were my motives in coming to Cuba? What was I going to do with the data I was collecting? I answered these questions with my usual research spiel, intentionally framing all of my answers to reflect the positive international reputation of the Cuban health care system. Criticizing anything, under the circumstances, seemed unwise.

Since the Revolution (I expounded authoritatively) Cuba had completely transformed its health indicators from Third World to First World levels. Health care in Cuba was freely available to everybody, while in the United States millions of poor people (including myself for several years) had no access to medical care whatsoever, and millions more suffered from preventable diseases or complications of existing conditions because their insurance companies or HMOs refused to authorize the necessary treatments. Yet despite the considerable economic and bureaucratic restrictions on access to quality medical care in the United States, health care costs as a whole were still spiraling out of control. Surely if the two systems were compared, the Cuban system (with its corresponding universal coverage and minimal costs) showed some notable superiorities.

My research project, as described in my original dissertation proposal (which, I reminded him, I had dutifully mailed to both the Cuban Interests Section in Washington, DC and the University of Havana), was motivated by a desire to see how the Cuban system worked first hand—to collect data on doctor-patient interactions and case studies that would allow me to offer a comprehensive micro-level portrayal of how Cuba's dramatic health care successes had come about. Furthermore, in addition to offering the Cubans a chance to publicize what was surely a great triumph of the Revolution, my research would simultaneously answer an ongoing theoretical debate within medical anthropology—the question of exactly *how* socialism transformed medical ideology and medical practice to bring about these population health improvements.

Brother Bob seemed more or less pleased with this response. He painstakingly noted down my statements word for word in a little notebook, leading me to wonder if perhaps the microphones in the room (and surely there must be microphones in the room) might (like every other piece of technical equipment in Cuba) be broken.

Brother Bob also seemed to perk up noticeably when I mentioned the importance of this research in configuring my future career options. "In the United States," I began, endeavoring to explain the requirements for a doctoral degree in anthropology, "all graduate students in cultural anthropology are expected to go to a foreign country for a year and do research for their doctoral thesis. If they are successful in their fieldwork, they can turn their thesis into a book, which is a big help as far as finding a job."

"Oh, so your research here is *very important for your career*," he mused with a noticeable glint in his eye, then began writing furiously in his notebook again. I went off on another long chatty spiel, all the while speculating in the back of my mind on why that particular bit of information would catch his attention so. Perhaps he was looking for points of leverage with me? If this research project was so important then maybe I could be induced to "help" them (whoever "they" were— certainly not the *Juventude*) in certain ways in exchange for permission to complete my study?

This was pure conjecture on my part, but it seemed like a reasonable guess. I didn't want to compromise myself ethically—no research project was important enough to risk surrendering myself to the dubious agenda of the Cuban secret police. In fact, I already felt like I was venturing into questionable terrain in that I was still steadfastly adhering to the enthusiastic adulation of my original research plan ("let me come and write about how wonderful your health care system is"), even though my months of residence in Cuba had already led me to suspect that a good deal of the famous revolutionary health care system was in actuality about as substantial as the castle at the center of Disney World—an impressive structure certainly, but one I suspected had been built primarily to be admired from afar.

At that particular moment, however, dropping my enthusiasm and publicly acknowledging doubts or criticizing the system would have certainly meant an immediate end to the project, which at the time seemed unthinkable. I had finally become acculturated to the point where I could linguistically navigate the dual worlds before me, and was able to use this newfound awareness to elicit a number of provocative and revealing narratives from people regarding their experiences with the system. People in the community had also become sufficiently accustomed to my presence that they no longer avoided talking about controversial subjects in front of me.

I had also stumbled upon a cache of uncatalogued and long-forgotten archival documents that painted a remarkably different historical picture of health trends in the pre-revolutionary era than I had ever encountered in any of the contemporary public health literature on Cuba. All of these data sources (historical and ethnographic) were beginning to coalesce into a pattern, but one I still felt powerless to fully conceptualize or understand. I was compelled, both out of intellectual curiosity, as well as a vague sense that I had stumbled onto to something important, to keep going as long as I was able.

As the interview was finally winding down, Brother Bob looked over and gave me one of his cold zealous smiles. "I have to go to Havana for a few days, so I'll give you a call when I get back and we can talk some more." He closed his notebook and looked over at me. "You know, Katherine," he intoned gravely, "I have so enjoyed our *intercambio* [interchange], and I just want you to know that if you ever need anything at all, you can feel free to ask me. The Juventude has power, you know, and we can help you. *We want to help you.* And while you're here in Santiago, I want you to think of me . . . I want you to think of me as part of your family—*like your brother.* "

I stifled a nervous laugh. How appropriate—my new (Orwellian) *Big Brother*. Who would no doubt always be watching me. With that the interview came to a close, silent Sister Cindy reappeared and together they drove me home in the battered little white Lada.

"So did you have a good time?" Lydia piped at me from the kitchen.

I said nothing and sat down in a rocking chair to collect myself. What in the world had just happened? The whole experience seemed surreal.

Lydia poked her head around from the kitchen. "Those people from the Juventude are nice, don't you think? It's good for you to be around young people for a change, instead of old ladies like me," she cackled a bit. "So, what did you do? Was there an *evento*?"

"Well, no . . . not exactly," I said slowly. "Actually, it was more in the way of an interrogation than an *evento*."

"Interrogation?" she exclaimed, startled.

"Well, they took me up to this house in Vista Allegre and sat me down alone in this little room and kept asking me questions about politics for about three hours. Lots of questions . . . "

"But what for?" she asked.

"For being American, I guess." I looked at her and shrugged. She looked back at me in tense silence. There seemed to be nothing else to say.

Over the next few days, I tried to dismiss my attacks of paranoia about the encounter with Brother Bob and Sister Cindy as a product of an overactive imagination. After all, nothing awful had happened—I was taken safely home with no problems. Most likely, I reasoned, the whole thing had just been a routine data-gathering interview as they began to compile a dossier on me. I had (again naively) assumed that the State Security would have been hard at work investigating me as far back as 1996 when I had first voiced a desire to do long-term field research in Cuba, but perhaps the police agencies were as vulnerable to the inefficiencies of the socialist system as all the other sectors. The whole experience had such an air of unreality to it in contrast to my previous experiences in Cuba at times I found myself doubting it ever really took place.

Not long after my first encounter with Brother Bob, I went to visit some friends in Santiago. At one point in the conversation, they (like many others before) began to caution me against "talking politics" with anyone on the street. "Don't ever," one of them said gravely, "talk about politics with *anyone*, no matter how trivial it might seem. Like if someone just sits down beside you on a bus or in a park or something and asks you about your political beliefs . . . " he trailed off.

"Oh, you know," I said with a puzzled laugh," something like that happened just the other day. Two people came to my house claiming to want some 'cultural interchange' with an American, and took me to a little room and asked me questions about my political beliefs for hours. Can you imagine a sillier pretense?" I chuckled sarcastically, "Like the next time I feel the need for some 'cultural interchange' with a Cuban I'll go grab one off the street, and take him to a little room in Vista Allegre and ask him questions about his political beliefs for hours . . . " I trailed off. They weren't laughing. In fact, it was hard not to notice that all the color had abruptly drained from their faces and they looked very noticeably afraid.

"Oh, Katherine," one of them whispered urgently, avoiding my gaze, "Please . . . You must be *very careful* with these people." Suddenly I felt a sharp resurgence of all the fear I had tried so hard to dismiss in the intervening days. The white Lada. The cold smiles. Perhaps my intuition of danger hadn't been so irrational after all.

Several days later, I had an appointment with a friend at the University who had been somewhat indirectly connected with my project. I instinctively trusted him, and since we were alone at the meeting I hesitantly mentioned my recent encounter with State Security. There was no mistaking the momentary flash of fear in his eyes. "*So they got you?*" he whispered incredulously, so low as to be practically inaudible.

I looked back at him. I had never anyone heard anyone speak of "Them" before. Like other happily oblivious visitors to Cuba before me, I had largely dismissed "Them" as figments of some old cold warrior's persecuted imagination. As Jorge Edwards (a Chilean diplomat stationed in Havana in the 1970s) stated before he realized the extent of the surveillance network in Cuba, "I had never seen the [state security] machine up close; therefore, I did not believe it was real" (1993:79). But suddenly, here "They" were—icons of the machine itself, manifest in the eerie persona of Brother Bob and inspiring such fear among my friends and acquaintances that "They" could only be spoken of in tense, fearful whispers. And somehow I had become of interest to "Them"—no doubt for some nefarious purpose I could hardly begin to imagine.

My friend quickly recovered his composure, then made a gesture that indicated it was unwise to talk of such things in the current surroundings.

"Look," he said, deliberately focusing his eyes away from the people on the periphery of the room, "Even now everyone is looking over here watching me talk to you. We should try and meet somewhere else . . . " He then suggested we arrange to meet "by accident" in a public spot downtown several days later where we could presumably talk for a few minutes without raising suspicions. It all seemed terribly cloak and dagger to me, but I agreed, curious to know what he had to say. I went to the arranged meeting place at the appointed time, but he failed to appear. Later I heard that he (like most everyone else I knew that week) had fallen sick with dengue.

Over the next few weeks, I was subject to further visits from Brother Bob. Curiously, he always seemed to know when to find me alone, making me wonder if he had secretly arranged with Lydia to get her out of the house beforehand. He continued his single-minded quest to elicit names of people I knew in the United Sates who were "similar to me"—progressive young people or academics who would be sympathetic to "the Revolution." "The Juventude," he assured me gravely, was actively campaigning with the Ministry of Public Health on my behalf so that I could finally get the health statistics I needed for my project. If I could just continue to help "the Revolution." One day he abruptly asked if he could borrow my address book and copy down all the names and phone numbers inside (I refused).

My last meeting with Brother Bob took place in mid June, and had a very different character from the previous meetings. He showed up at the house midmorning (curiously enough, once again when Lydia had gone out on an errand) and began immediately quizzing me on various aspects of political theory. What were my thoughts on the fall of the Soviet Union? I remember feeling quite irritated by this line of questioning—it was terribly hot that day, and I was still fatigued from my bout of dengue, and had no desire to expend my limited strength discussing global politics. I mumbled some incoherent phrases and tried to turn the tables by asking him some questions in return. Brother Bob had a passion for oratory and began expounding at length on all kinds of subjects, allowing me the luxury of escaping into a restful waking nap. He droned on for some time.

At one point though, I became aware of a sudden silence. I refocused my gaze and saw was looking at me expectantly. "I'm sorry," I apologized, hoping to politely extricate myself. "I'm not sure I understand . . . " He began another long, circuitous narrative, obliquely mentioning that a group of American students was expected in Santiago later that month as part of a summer school program. After much conversational back and forth, I finally caught on that he was asking me if I would "get close to" this group of students and provide him with a report of the ideological position and political beliefs of everyone in the group.

"Aha!" I exclaimed, with just the right amount of conspiratorial enthusiasm, "You want me to *infiltrate* this group of American students—like a spy!"

My goal in forcing the issue this way was to gain some rhetorical advantage for myself by forcing him to overtly confirm or deny what he seemed to be asking me to do—in other words to strip away the veil of secrecy he was trying so hard to maintain. (As Solzhenitsyn once noted, "They [i.e., State Security] can't *work* in the public eye" (1973:16)—meaning that secrecy and doublespeak are essential components of "their" power.) If Brother Bob admitted what he was asking me to do, (i.e., by stating "Yes, I want you to spy on this group of students and report back to me") then he would be essentially acknowledging the dark depravity of his agenda, not to mention the "The Revolution's" deep and unending paranoia. If he denied it, of course, (i.e., by stating, "No, of course I don't want you to spy on these students") I would presumably be off the hook.

Somewhat to his credit (and much to my surprise), instead of answering the question, Brother Bob simply burst out laughing. And then, in a response that perplexes me still, he looked up (still chuckling) and said, "Ah, Katherine . . . sometimes I have a hard time believing you aren't Cuban!" I assume, given the extreme xenophobia that characterizes most Cuban State Security, that this was intended to be some kind of compliment, but one I remain powerless to fully understand.

Then, he simply began reiterating his original dark circumlocutions, arguing with great intensity that my participation in this (nameless) endeavor would be highly desirable for all concerned. "No." I interrupted. "I won't do it."

He looked vaguely offended, and began yet another series of arguments. "You can keep talking all morning," I said wearily, "but you're not going to change my mind." With that I knew it was all over. I had become uncooperative. I was sure my research visa would be revoked in the upcoming weeks.

But Brother Bob was still not quite finished though. He paused for a moment and appeared to mentally shift gears. "So tell me, Mary," he began, "does anyone in your family work for the United States government?" I looked back at him, puzzled.

"Um . . . I have an uncle that was in the Air Force, but he's retired now," I said hesitantly, "And anyway, I hardly even know him." What in the world could he be getting at now, asking about my family?

Brother Bob's face remained inscrutable. He paused for a moment. "Would you mind if someone contacted you in the United States in my name?" he asked suddenly.

What was this!? I had a momentary nightmarish vision of mysterious Cubans knocking on my door in the dark of night whispering, "José-Carlos sent me . . . "

"I would prefer not," I said, as politely as I could manage under the circumstances. With that the interview was over. About two weeks later, the University abruptly declared that unless I immediately paid my entire "research fee" in full, immediately, they would be forced to revoke my visa and I would not be allowed to stay in Cuba. I reluctantly (though not without some measure of relief) began making plans to go home early.

Disintegration

It felt terrible to contemplate going home so soon. There was still so much left to do, and I knew once I left I there would be no coming back. Plus I had grown so close to Lydia and my other friends that I became wracked with survivor's guilt. It seemed wrong that I could use a Get Out of Jail Free Card to end my Cuba ordeal while they were forced to stay behind. I also knew that exercising my freedom to leave would make me the object of considerable envy—envy that would destroy or at least diminish a good deal of the rapport I had been building over the past seven months.

Up to that point I had willingly foregone the perks Cuba awards to foreigners. I waited in food lines, rarely shopped at dollar stores and took public transportation. My clothes were worn from the sun and the rough laundry soap, and I often looked much shabbier than my Cuban friends, who (despite considerable material deprivation) managed to remain very fashionable. The fact that I did not engage in the kind of conspicuous consumption associated with most foreign travelers in Cuba meant that I had gained some measure of acceptance in the community. As one neighbor stated, "Cubans are funny. If they think you have less than they do they are the most generous people in the world. They'll take you in and give you everything. But if they think you have more than they do and aren't sharing, they'll be relentless about trying to take advantage of you." I felt fortunate that I was legitimately poor enough during most of my stay to avoid at least some of the resentment that foreigners endured. But now, reminding people that I could leave Cuba whenever I wanted while they had to stay behind seemed the worst flaunting of wealth I could have done.

Other factors also compelled me to end my fieldwork early. At the time of my arrival, it was still permissible for Cubans to rent rooms to visiting tourists and it was not illegal for me to privately contract with Lydia for room and board. The state did not encourage these kinds of activities, but seemed willing to tolerate them due to the fact that hotel construction was lagging behind consumer demand and there was an ongoing shortage of rooms. Starting in the summer of 1997, however, (and coinciding with the completion of a number of new hotels) a series of increasingly restrictive laws were enacted designed to limit Cubans' participation in the informal market in tourist services and to heavily police the ability of ordinary Cubans to interact with foreigners. Called the "Campaign Against Indiscipline and Inefficiency" it was widely publicized in Cuban newspapers such as *Granma*, *Juventude Rebelde,* and *Trabajadores*.

The Campaign Against Indiscipline condemned individuals engaged in black or grey market activities (such as renting rooms to foreigners) as counterrevolutionaries, and called upon organizations such as the CDR to aggressively police their neighborhoods to stamp out these criminal behaviors. The newspaper *Trabajadores*, for instance, ran an editorial on April 18, 1997 that read, "Nothing threatens us more today than these outbreaks of laziness, irresponsibility and corruption. Like crime and illegality, they are equivalent to a perpetual invasion by the enemy."

The more extremist newspaper of Oriente province, *Sierra Maestra*, actually insinuated that these acts of economic indiscipline (i.e. undermining state control of the economy) were the local equivalent of an imperialist plot to destroy the revolution. On June 21, 1997 an editorial stated, "These social indisciplines embody a great danger for the survival of the Revolution, and play into the hands of imperialists who seek to destroy us, to liquidate and subvert us by making us weak and divided." Increased neighborhood surveillance was justified with the argument that it was necessary to go backwards (to the more repressive days of the 1960s) in order to gain the momentum to leap forward (presumably into a utopian future). *Granma*, for instance, defended the campaign against indiscipline as "the only way [for the revolution] to come out definitively ahead" (May 3, 1997).

The effects of these policies were immediate and severe. Before the Campaign Against Indiscipline began, a steady stream of black marketeers appeared at the house every day offering a variety of foods for sale at discount prices. Enterprising produce vendors also purchased fruits and vegetables at the farmers markets in the morning and roamed the streets throughout the day, reselling at a slight markup to elderly women who had no transportation to the market. Several other families in the neighborhood rented rooms to foreign tourists.

Given the intensity of the economic crisis in Santiago, almost everyone was forced to rely on the black market for such vital necessities as eggs, flour, chicken, milk, coffee, cheese and meat. Even commodities as basic as table salt could be difficult to obtain in the peso economy. The possibility of being penalized for buying these meager essentials on the black market threw everyone into a quiet uproar, and many saw it as a blatant attempt to force them to purchase their foods in the costly *diplotiendas*. One man described deep disgust with these developments, yet felt powerless to voice any dissent at the meeting. "I had to stay quiet," he sighed morosely, "otherwise they'll report that I'm not showing the proper revolutionary spirit."

By early June the flow of black market and produce vendors had all but stopped. The few that did appear told tales of being waylaid and searched by the police on their way into the city. Often they had their contraband seized and significant fines imposed. One woman from whom I bought a chicken wearily described how she was forced to increase her black market sales in order to make enough money to pay the fines she had already incurred. Another neighbor told of having agents from the Ministry of the Interior arrive at her house and forcibly evict two Canadian tourists who were renting rooms from her.

Policemen were stationed on every block in heavily touristed areas, and police patrols increased dramatically along beaches and in nightclubs. If a Cuban was observed talking with or approaching a foreigner, he or she would be detained and arrested. This was ostensibly to protect tourists from petty theft and harassment from *jiniteras*. Many people I spoke with, however, were quite cynical of these stated motives and instead believed the crackdown was a move by the state to enforce its monopoly on tourist services by arresting those who attempt to undersell it in the informal economy. *Jiniteros* frequently served as informal conduits that redirected foreign visitors (and their hard currency) away from expensive state restaurants and hotels and into paladares and private homes.

By late summer large yellow school buses and military trucks were stationed near key tourist areas. Police scoured surrounding blocks, randomly checking identity cards of anyone who looked like they might be *jiniteando*. Those with suspect work histories or previous offenses written on their *carnet de identidad* were hauled away to the buses, and at the end of the day they were all taken to a central processing area where they were assessed hefty fines. These buses were also known to circulate through touristed areas late at night rounding up prostitutes—sometimes as many as two or three hundred in a single sweep.

In early June, a neighborhood CDR meeting was convened to discuss the Campaign Against Indiscipline. By that point I had learned that the purpose of these kinds of meetings was not to "discuss" new policies but to reinforce them. No one was allowed to question the policies themselves. As a foreigner I couldn't attend the meeting myself, but the events that transpired there became the subject of neighborhood gossip for many weeks. According to several reports, neighborhood residents were singled out during this meeting for their assorted acts of indiscipline (such as buying food on the black market or renting rooms to tourists) and warned that if they didn't desist, penalties or fines would be incurred. Furthermore, these individuals were expected to publicly acknowledge their wrongdoing at the meeting, regardless of the fact that these activities had previously been considered acceptable and were often necessary for survival.

My presence in Lydia's house did not escape notice. It was later reported to me that the head of the vigilance committee in the CDR looked around the room and demanded of the assembled participants, "And what are we going to about this AMERICAN living in our neighborhood?!" The message was clear—whereas before I had been welcome as a friend and visitor, this change in policy meant I had become a political liability. Much to their dismay, my friends and neighbors were now collectively required to denounce my presence as an act of neighborhood indiscipline. If I wanted to stay in Santiago, I would have to move into a hotel to spare Lydia further CDR persecution. The woman who described these events to me was furious,

> My husband was such a good communist he gave away all his salary and left me nothing. Not even a color TV. And this witch [the CDR vigilance committee chair] is trying to put people down for having foreigners! My husband was a real communist, not a thief or a shameless hustler or a snitch like these people. He left me nothing. And now she has the nerve to criticize us for [things like] this?!

She had a point. Her husband (who had passed away in 1995) had been a devout, altruistic communist who had freely given away his salary. The state had at various times rewarded his loyalty with such commodities as a Lada and a black and white television, but beyond these meager possessions she had very little.

Many people expressed similar outrage at the duplicity of the economic crackdown, particularly the double standard that seemed to prevail for those with political connections. But no one would speak out. If people had stated their true feelings at the meeting, they would have likely received red marks on their employment history record, or possibly even lost their jobs altogether. Given the complete state control of the economy, unemployment would have likely been a permanent condition, requiring complete dependency on the earnings and good will of his family members. The overwhelming economic difficulties most families faced made political dissent an unaffordable luxury.

A new housing law was also passed as part of the Campaign Against Indiscipline. This law was intended to legalize the common practice of renting rooms to foreign tourists by imposing a tax on those who engage in this activity. In actuality, the effect of this legislation was the opposite of its stated intention—the taxes were so high and inflexible that most people were forced to abandon renting altogether. Two hundred and fifty American dollars had to be paid to the state for each room rented, per month, regardless of whether or not the rental units were occupied. A percentage of gross revenues was assessed at the end of every fiscal year as well. No food could be provided, or else a fine would be incurred.

Those found to be renting illegally were assessed a U.S. $400 fine for the first offense. Subsequent offenses were penalized by confiscation of the house itself. According to informal reports from Havana, Ministry of the Interior agents soon began a methodical campaign to entrap illegal renters by impersonating foreign tourists.

The change in the housing law seemed to seal my fate. I could stay at Lydia's for another month, but after that I would have to move. I hated the thought of living in a sterile hotel. Despite a number of joint economic ventures, the tourism industry in Cuba was still run on the principles of monopoly capitalism, and even cheap hotels were often low quality and outrageously expensive. Plus it was well known that most hotels were staffed with State Security agents. These jobs were considered rewards for the politically loyal—it gave them high-paying tourism jobs, access to scarce luxury supplies such as soap and shampoo (which they could steal and sell on the black market), as well as an opportunity to spy on foreign visitors and businessmen. No, it would be much better to go home for a while than move to a hotel.

Another reason I knew I should consider an early departure was that I was increasingly unable to cope with the various stresses in my life. Heat, sun, illness, isolation, and constant harassment by *jiniteros*, plus the lurking presence of Brother Bob all combined to fray my nerves well beyond the breaking point. But still it wasn't easy. When I told Lydia, her face fell, and my heart broke.

"When will you go?" she asked plaintively.

"Maybe a month. And then I'll try and come back again in a few more months." I tried to sound positive but my words felt hollow. Even if I did come back, I wouldn't be able to live with her anyway.

"Well, I guess it's for the best," she said, trying hard to put a cheerful spin on things. "We'll give you a big *despedida* [going away party]." But something vital began to ebb from our relationship.

It didn't take long for word of my departure to spread. People were good sports about it, but the envy was palpable. One of the doctors I worked with drifted into a dreamy reverie over the wonders of travel,

"I love Cuba," she sighed. "And I would never want to live anywhere else, but still . . . to travel, how beautiful."

"Where would you want to go?" I asked her.

"Oh, I imagine myself traveling all over the world, learning about other people, other customs. But always coming back to Cuba. I would never want to leave my country. But still, here it's impossible [to travel abroad]. Last week I was on vacation, and you know where I went? Home. And to visit my husband's family in Guantanamo. Now what kind of a vacation is that?"

She paused with a faraway look on her face. "Oh, I'd love so love to go to Brazil. I saw this Brazilian on the street the other day and he was so beautiful I just walked by him and stared. Then I blurted out, '*Oh, Dios mio*' right to him before I realized what I was doing!" At the point we both dissolved into laughter at her indiscretion. "Oh, but I'm just dreaming," she said, shaking her head. "I'll travel in my dreams."

My suspicions about the legitimacy of Cuba's health claims deepened further when I went to visit the officials at the University of the Oriente to complete the paperwork necessary for my departure. Dr. Supervisor did not seem sorry to see me go. He simply shrugged and said, "It's true that public health here is *bien cerrada* [very closed.]" I was momentarily taken aback. Nothing I had ever read in the United States implied that the Cubans were closed or secretive about their health system. In fact, other researchers had praised the openness and accuracy of Cuba's health statistics (see Feinsilver, 1993; Santana, 1988).

Another professor I had worked with was standing in the doorway to Dr. Supervisor's office at the time. He suddenly began chastising me. "You know you can't just show up at the public health office alone, unaccompanied. Of course they're not going to believe you [are who you say you are]. And some of those statistics are classified anyway. No one can seen them."

This was also news. Health statistics in Cuba were classified secrets? I sensed by the obfuscation I had encountered in the local Ministry of Health that they were reluctant to share information, but this was the first time I had heard mention of health indicators being considered state secrets. Yet they couldn't be too classified since the central MINISAP office in Havana freely handed out compilations of national health statistics to anyone who requested them. Unless, of course, those statistics were false, and the true disease rates were kept under lock and key. Many people in Santiago told me they suspected the dengue outbreak was kept secret because publicity might hurt tourism revenues. If that were the case, it seemed likely that rates of STDs and HIV in Cuba were also much higher than the reported figures since sex tourism and prostitution had become such key revenue producers in Cuba's new economy. I couldn't help but wonder if all disease rates that might reflect negatively on the Cuban government were being kept secret.

"And why are health statistics kept classified?" I asked innocently. Now that Dr. Supervisor had admitted this duplicity, I was curious to see how he would justify it. Surely he wouldn't admit that releasing honest statistics might embarrass the government. But what other explanation could there be?

"Because other people have come here seeking to do harm to *nuestra revolución!*" Dr. Supervisor thundered, stabbing the air with his index finger in a gesture remarkably reminiscent of Fidel in a fit of revolutionary fervor.

I had to stifle a laugh. It was an absurd answer, but very revealing of the logic (or strategic illogic) of the Cuban system. I knew the irrationality of his statement would be lost on him—Cuba did not train people to think critically about official pronouncements, only to repeat them with tremendous fervor. But to me, a dangerous independent thinker, Dr. Supervisor's statement meant that any facts that might discredit the Castro regime were quite likely kept secret and/or denounced as the work of enemy sabateurs. Later, after my return to the United States I ran across a quote from a former Soviet dissident who stated, "It [socialism] is a world of appearances trying to pass for reality . . . because the regime is captive to its own lies, it must falsify everything" (quoted in Gleason, 1997:185). It certainly seemed to explain a lot about Cuba.

As the date of my departure grew near a number of new crises suddenly hit. The day before my flight, a neighbor came by and breathlessly informed me that the daily plane from Santiago to Havana (the same flight I was scheduled to take the next day) had crashed, killing everyone on board. People at the airport claimed the plane exploded, but the Cuban government released little information other than stating it was an accident, not a deliberate attack. Forty-four people died, including eight foreign tourists.

A phone call from Havana brought more bad news—the city was under terrorist attack. Several bombs had gone off in tourist hotels, and a visiting Italian had been killed. If that wasn't enough to make my departure sufficiently stressful, I also had word from a local doctor that Santiago was experiencing an outbreak of a particularly incapacitating flu virus, and a major epidemic of hemorrhagic conjunctivitis was underway in Havana. Hemorrhagic conjunctivitis is an extremely contagious disease, and while not fatal, usually leaves its victims immobilized for about two weeks, with eyeballs painfully swollen to horrific proportions.

I finished packing my bags wondering which of these dreadful catastrophes was likely to befall me next. At the very least, I sighed, it would feel good to get out of Santiago, even if it was on an exploding airplane. Part of me was still fatalistically convinced I was destined to die in Cuba.

My plane didn't blow up, but I did wake up with a terrific case of flu the next morning. There are few things in life more unpleasant that the first day of a bad flu. When one has to rise at dawn, say tearful goodbyes to cherished friends one will almost certainly never see again, get on an aged (and potentially exploding) Air Cubana jet destined for a potentially exploding Havana hotel, the awfulness is particularly acute. Even though it was early in the morning when I boarded the plane I tearfully sipped a flask of rum until my agonies subsided.

I spent five uncomfortable days in Havana recuperating at the Hotel Ambos Mundos, where I inadvertently infected at least half of the staff and probably several of the other guests with my aggressive *grippe Oriental*. I had given away almost all of my medicines before I left Santiago, and was forced to take an expensive taxi to the international clinic in Miramar and pay U.S. $25 (a full month's wages for a family doctor in Santiago) to a very aged and nearsighted physician in order to get a prescription for lozenges and cough medicine.

As I waited in line at the dollar pharmacy the contradictions of Cuba's economy again struck me full force. There were no medications of any sort—not even aspirin or band-aids—available in the peso economy, yet the dollar pharmacies were amply supplied. So many North American medical journals (including the prestigious *American Journal of Public Health*) decried the U.S trade embargo as "immoral" (http://www.slu.edu/publications/ge/v6–9/news_17.shtml), a form of "child abuse" (Kirkpatrick, 2002) or even "genocide" because it imposed restrictions on food and medications. But the well-stocked dollar pharmacies suggested there was no problem importing medicines to sell for profit. It was only the peso sector of the economy that was so impoverished. Given that both the peso and the dollar pharmacies were operated by same the government, I suspected that the Cubans were just trying to maximize revenues by selling medications for dollars instead of dispensing them for free through the public sector.

Part Two

History Revisited

5

Reframing History

The experience of conducting long-term fieldwork in Cuba completely discredited the Marxist model of political economy and health for me. The body of research that originally framed my dissertation research proposal seemed to explain nothing about the reality of everyday life in my study communities. Why was there no mention of Cuba's stifling bureaucracy, repression, political corruption and widespread popular cynicism? Why did scholarship in medical anthropology focus only on health statistics, and exclude any critical discussion of the authoritarian measures (including imprisonment of dissident doctors) by which those statistics were produced?

In my own case, the experience of living everyday life in Cuba—confronting the thousands of petty humiliations, harassments, artificial commodity shortages and official lies one must endure to simply survive—left me unable to sustain any belief in the Marxist ideal of socialism. The reality was simply too unpleasant. As it turns out, this intellectual path is well traveled. A number of foreign visitors and scholars who have spent time in Cuba (including several Marxists and noted ex-Marxists) have written powerful critiques of the socialist regime (see Corbett, 2002; Daniels, 1991; Duberman, 1975; Edwards, 1993; Halperin, 1994; Radosh, 2001; Timmerman, 1990; Lewis, 1977; Hollander, 1998; Dumont, 1974). Many former Cuban dissidents and revolutionaries (and their family members) have also authored critical exposés about their experiences with the revolutionary government (see Betancourt, 2001; Montaner, 1981; Montaner, 1985; Llovio-Menendez, 1988; Franqui, 1985; Fernández, 1997; Masetti, 1993; Valladares, 1986). And some of Cuba's most gifted writers have penned disturbing narratives of ideological coercion and violence at the hands of revolutionary officials (see Arenas, 1993; 1994; Cabrera-Infante, 1994; Padilla, 1984; Montaner, 1981).

There is a curious myopia within anthropology, however, that has largely excluded these critical voices from intellectual discourse in the profession. A few anthropologists have published accounts of field research on the island that detail difficult and unpleasant encounters with Cuban state security officials (see Lewis, 1977; Rosendahl, 1997). In the case of Oscar Lewis (who began his research project at the personal invitation of Fidel Castro), authorities abruptly revoked his research permission, expelled him from the country, denounced him as a "counterrevolutionary," and arrested at least one of his informants who had criticized the regime. These narratives, however, have had relatively little impact on Cuba's image in most anthropological scholarship, which continues to be favorable or neutral.

After I returned from Cuba, I discovered a number of other graduate students in the social sciences working on the island in the late 1990s also had negative experiences with Cuban authorities. While some people had no problems and thoroughly enjoyed their research experiences, others reported various forms of bureaucratic and political harassment, ranging from mild to severe. One student was expelled from the country with no explanation. Nearly all complained of political intrusion into their research, and attempts by Cuban officials to control their access to research materials. Despite these difficulties, however, no one was willing to publicly criticize the Cuban government for its treatment of foreign researchers, or bring these issues to the attention of professional groups such as the Latin American Studies Association or the American Anthropological Association. Some students feared Cuban officials might exact retribution against their trusted friends and *socios* on the island. Others were afraid of losing access to their research sites, and a few voiced concerns about the professional marginalization that would result if they were to become perceived as ideologically conservative. One student experienced pressure from her dissertation advisor to keep quiet, out of fear that he would subsequently lose access to his research community in Cuba.

All of these concerns are legitimate. In the early 1990s, a group of faculty members at the University of Havana were fired for making indiscreet comments to foreign researchers. Several North American academics who wrote very *uncritical* books about the Castro regime remain barred from further research on the island for expressing minor deviations from the Party Line. Scholars in the United States who have written critical works on Cuba, or who have publicly voiced disappointment with the regime still endure painful attacks from leftist colleagues and marginalization from mainstream academic discourse (see Radosh, 2001; Duberman, 1975; Hollander, 1998; Montaner, 1981).

In other words, the difficulties associated with anthropological research in Cuba do not stop with the termination of one's fieldwork. Writing up research results also presents a number of challenges. Is it wrong to present a singularly distorted and positive image of life in Cuba, if doing so protects trusted informants and *socios* from political retribution? How much liberty can one take with ethnographic data to disguise informants without "fictionalizing?" At what point does concealing expressions of political dissent become self-censorship?

Contemporary ethnography has ostensibly moved away from the univocal (and presumably hegemonic) narratives of the past, and into a new genre characterized by an emphasis on polyphony and reflexivity (see Clifford, 2002). Such an approach, however, is still not possible in the case of Cuba. As long as public dissent from the regime remains a crime, critical voices must be erased or distorted in anthropological writing. The ethnographic texts that result from these endeavors thus become complicit in the regime's censorship and suppression of dissent.[1] In the case of Cuba, it is the dissidents who are the real subaltern, yet their voices have been most profoundly excluded from anthropological writings.

In my own case, I did not want to put my friends or myself at risk by writing an ethnographic text that would incorporate all of the criticisms and "counterrevolutionary" sentiments I encountered in my study communities. But I was also unwilling to erase these voices, or surrender my own subjective opinions to better fit in with the decidedly uncritical writings in mainstream anthropology. The historical material presented in the succeeding chapters is intended as something of a compromise between these conflicting agendas—a way to maintain a critical perspective and validate the complaints of Cuban dissidents, without revealing confidential information that would endanger individual informants.

An Alternative History

The remaining chapters of this work offer a revisionist health history of twentieth century Cuba. This history is intended to critique the conventional portrayal of these events by the Castro regime and by Marxist scholars in the United States. To elaborate, the Castro revolutionaries have always invoked a rhetoric of historical messianism to justify their monopolization of power since 1959. Key elements of this narrative include the reconfiguration of time itself to reflect a new beginning of history. In keeping with this temporal arrangement, the years from 1902–1959 are collapsed into a single "pre-Revolutionary" period, ostensibly characterized by suffering, exploitation and disease at the hands of Yankee imperialists and dictators such as Fulgencio Batista. The 1959 revolution is then portrayed as a pivotal event that effectively saved Cuba from the violent depredations of the United States, restored the island's health and well-being and brought about the successful realization of José Martí's nationalist vision. The following excerpt from a 1997 newspaper article in Santiago neatly encapsulates this narrative, and frames the 1959 revolution and the transition to communism as the living embodiment of José Martí's ideals,

From the first Cuban independence struggles, the principal strategic enemy of our sovereignty has been the expansionists and annexationists in the United States government. In 1898 this crime against our independence was consummated. Marti and Maceo had died, and they came to the moment to execute their dark ambitions. It [the Spanish-American War] was an annexationist war against Cuban independence. Cuba had to suffer six decades of neocolonization before the triumph of 1959. . . . As such, the grand achievements of our pueblo in the Great War, the Second War of Independence and the War of Liberation that culminated in the victory of January 1959 are inseparable parts of the same Revolution. The cries of 'Independence or Death," "Liberty or Death," "Fatherland or Death," and "Socialism or Death" are expressions of a historical continuum. Symbols of glory. The Monroe Doctrine, the [U.S. military] Intervention in 1898, the Platt Amendment, the Blockade [the U.S. trade embargo], the Torrecelli and Helmes-Burton Laws are also a historical continuum. Symbols of ignominy. Today in this scenario of struggle, the same forces converge. The reactionaries, that from [Thomas] Jefferson to [Bill] Clinton are enemies of our independence and fight to deprive us of it. And those revolutionaries that from [Carlos Manuel de] Cespedes to Fidel defend this independence with the conviction to never lose it. The lesson of history is clear. There is only one Revolution that we are building and defending. One enemy that we combat and conquer (Molina, 1997).

As previously mentioned, a number of contemporary researchers in medical anthropology and public health have maintained a leftist or dependency perspective that uncritically reiterates key features of this historical narrative. Most medical anthropologists and Marxist historians, for instance, speak as if there was only one Cuban revolution in the twentieth century. In reality, the years between 1902 and 1959 saw an almost constant succession of revolutionary movements and insurrections. There were at least ten major insurrections and four successful revolutions prior to 1959. When elections were held during these years, they were often accompanied by gunfights and political assassinations. According to most observers at the time, this turbulence was not produced by class struggle against enemy imperialists, but by rival *caudillo* factions seeking access to the economic spoils of power.

Warfare has always been a key factor in precipitating disease outbreaks, as subsistence activities and nutrition become compromised by violence, loss of infrastructure, and diversion of key resources to armies. The near constant instability of Cuba's republican years would have been sufficient to interfere with health programs and disease eradication efforts. When the destructive cycles of graft and political corruption in the various governments are added to this equation, it is not difficult to see how infectious diseases continued to thrive in Cuba during these years.

The following chapters will present an alternative health history for Cuba from the end of the War of Independence (1898) until the Castro revolution of 1959. Rather than dismissing this time period as a single "pre-Revolutionary" era, this history will explore Cuba's political violence and instability, as well as associated graft and corruption in the public health sector. In some ways this history is incomplete—it focuses almost entirely on violence and corruption in the public sector and often neglects to explore the actions and activities of foreign capitalists in Cuba.

The reasons for this focus have to do in part with the nature of disease transmission. Infectious diseases tend to proliferate where drinking water is contaminated by sewage or other pathogens, where insects or rodents can multiply unchecked near human habitations, and where large numbers of people live in crowded conditions, without resources or access to adequate nutrition. In urban areas, control over these key components of environmental health typically rests with municipal health and sanitation programs, not private physicians or foreign corporations. In some cases, public officials may react defensively if international entities such as corporations or NGOs attempt to take on these responsibilities themselves. Failure of public health and sanitation efforts can often have catastrophic consequences—high population densities in urban areas (especially if large numbers of people are poorly nourished) mean any outbreak of disease can readily become amplified into a major epidemic. In rural areas, where government services do not exist, disease vectors often proliferate unchecked. This neglect is rarely as grave as in urban areas, however, since low population densities and lack of sophisticated transportation networks in rural areas can be sufficient to keep outbreaks of infectious disease localized.

Conventional scholarship linking imperialism with ill health often fails to identify the specific process by which increasing foreign control of a nation's economy contributes to the amplification of pathogens in rural or urban environments. These arguments are instead based largely on historical correlation: poor health indicators occurred simultaneously with increasing North American control of the Cuban economy, so U.S. capitalism is assumed to be responsible. This argument however, confuses correlation with causation, and fails to address the key importance of the local public health infrastructure in identifying and controlling disease vectors.

If U.S. imperialism were truly the root cause of Cuba's ill health and underdevelopment prior to 1959, then it would be logical to expect archival evidence to reveal examples of U.S. corporations pressuring local and national political leaders to cut or minimize health and sanitation programs. If Cuban leaders defied these demands, archival records should reveal U.S. officials forcing Cuban leaders to follow the dictates of capitalists and foreign corporations. In actuality, archival evidence supports a very different scenario. Historical records in Cuba and in the United States suggest that the United States exerted imperial political pressure on Cuba's leaders to *improve* local health conditions, since epidemics of infectious disease were both bad for business, and a threat to southern port cities in the United States.

Sugar mills, copper mines and other industrial factories require a steady supply of healthy workers. High rates of worker absenteeism due to infectious diseases such as yellow fever or malaria was often viewed as a significant deterrent to the optimal functioning of capitalist enterprises in Cuba in the early 1900s. As a result, both U.S. corporations and the U.S. government sought to improve health conditions in Cuba. In urban areas such as Havana and Santiago, the United States tried to engineer the construction of major public works projects (such as waterworks, sewer systems and roads) that would prevent disease outbreaks. These efforts were frequently stymied by local and national politicians intent on co-opting public funds for themselves. Even political pressure by the imperial power was often insufficient to overcome this local resistance. As a result, Havana's water supply remained contaminated for many years, and annual typhoid epidemics continued unabated.

In rural areas, U.S. corporations also tried a variety of programs to reduce worker absenteeism due to infectious disease. In some cases, these were coercive programs designed to force unhealthy workers to perform their jobs regardless (as in the "company doctor" pattern described by rural mine workers in the United States). In other cases, legitimate health improvement efforts were undertaken. One U.S. mining company in Oriente Province, for instance, boasted of having reduced worker absenteeism from malaria by almost one hundred percent between 1901 and 1909 through stringent mosquito control measures (Lindsey, 1911). Even if these improvements were motivated primarily by economic considerations, they still resulted in important health gains for workers.

Some scholars have argued that imperialism produces ill health by increasing poverty and inequality in a given locale. There is some validity to these claims. Poverty has always been an overwhelmingly important variable in configuring outbreaks of infectious disease (see McKeown, 1976; Farmer, 1999; 1994). Poverty, however, is not produced by imperialism alone. Unequal taxes imposed by local elites can also dramatically increase the burden of low wages and poor nutrition on workers. In the case of Cuba (and many other Latin American republics during the twentieth century), the public sector has always been exceptionally parasitic. Tax burdens were shifted disproportionately to the poor, and taxes were used to fund vastly overgrown militaries and government bureaucracies that provided little in the way of useful services to the population. Avaricious dictators also helped themselves liberally to public revenues (see Andreski, 1966).

In Cuba rival out-of-power political groups also imposed their own informal taxes on the population through various extortion activities. Competing revolutionary groups earned money to buy weapons through kidnapping, smuggling and extorting funds from legitimate businesses. These activities, combined with the parasitic tax structure of the regular government imposed a tremendous economic burden on Cuban workers as well as on capitalists. In 1910, Irene Wright (p. 160) described the Cuban government as, "the most expensive government on earth," and noted that, "those who operate it (the Cuban office-holding class) have every reason to labor to make it even more so, since its extravagances run to salaries, which they receive . . . " During this time, nearly eighty-five percent of state funds were generated from customs revenues, which were steadily increased to support the growing extravagance of government officials. Given that Cuba imported nearly all of its basic foodstuffs, this amounted to a massive form of hidden taxation, leveled equally upon the wealthy as the poor, for basic necessities of life. Under these circumstances, is it realistic to assert that the plight of the poor in Cuba resulted solely from North American imperialism? Or should the relationship between poverty and disease be viewed as involving number of diverse variables, including the parasitic nature of the Cuban government and the neglect of basic public health prevention measures by political officials?

The minimization of the U.S. economic presence in Cuba in the subsequent chapters of this work is not intended to disparage its significance. Instead, this approach is intended to highlight the significance of these other, often-overlooked variables (such as the parasitic nature of the public sector, and the ongoing *caudillo*-driven violence and instability) in configuring the relationship between poverty and disease in Cuba prior to 1959.

This historical material is presented chronologically. Chapter 6 begins with a discussion of health conditions during the Spanish-Cuban-American War, emphasizing the dramatic turnaround in health conditions that took place from 1898–1906. During this time, infectious diseases such as typhoid, yellow fever and malaria became effectively controlled due to the stringent (and repressive) health and sanitation programs put in place during the U.S. military occupation of Cuba.

Chapters seven and eight explore how factionalism and *caudillismo* led to health declines and additional U.S. intervention under the Platt Amendment during the early years of the republic. Chapters nine and ten explore how international criminal syndicates merged with Cuba's corrupt political elites (including officials in the Ministry of Health) in the 1940s and 1950s in ways that further exacerbated problems of infection control and infrastructure decline in Cuba's major cities.

A Note on Sources

This alternative historical narrative necessarily privileges certain sources of information over others. It is assumed, for instance, that Cuba's early political leaders would seek to minimize public awareness of their own appropriation of public funds, while exaggerating the misconduct of their rivals. These dual patterns of secrecy and exaggeration make accurate historical investigation of corruption in Cuba difficult—narratives from any Cuban political leaders that reveal or deny misconduct or personal appropriation of funds must be viewed with some skepticism.

This history is also biased toward North American rather than Cuban archival sources. During my original field research in Cuba in the late 1990s, I was given permission to use the provincial archives in the city of Santiago, as well as the reading library in the Carlos Finlay Museum in Havana. Officials at the national archives in Havana, however, would not allow me access to their collections. Fortunately, there are a number of North American sources that detail events and conditions in Cuba during the first half of the twentieth century. The United States Public Health Service maintained an office in Cuba from the late 1800s until the mid-1930s. In addition to data on communicable diseases, these USPHS reports often included descriptions of various political and military activities on the island, as well as occasional critiques of U.S. policies on the island.

During the second U.S. military occupation of the island (from 1906–1909) U.S. army personnel sent confidential reports to Charles Magoon (the provisional governor) describing the actions and activities of local political groups, with corresponding discussions of how these individuals were likely to respond to the political agenda of the U.S. occupying army. These reports also describe the political difficulties faced by U.S. army personnel in attempting to undertake public works and public health improvements on the island—local officials in some provinces apparently believed that distributing public works sinecures was their domain, and at times sought to derail health programs mandated by the provisional governor. These criticisms were echoed in correspondence sent from local Cuban health and sanitation officials to their superiors in Havana and in Washington, DC.

Several journalists and historians also described these dynamics in the early twentieth century. Charles Chapman's (1927) *A History of the Cuban Republic* remains the most comprehensive secondary source detailing Cuba's early political corruption and violence. Journalists Irene Wright and Ruby Hart Phillips were both astute (and critical) observers of Cuban social and political life. Leading Cuban intellectuals such as Emilio Roig de Leuschenring (1924) and Fernando Ortiz (1929) published exposés denouncing graft and political corruption as a legacies of Spanish colonialism. Health and sanitation were also frequent themes in State Department correspondence between the United States and Cuba throughout the first half of the twentieth century.

During the 1920s and early 1930s, the U.S. Coast Guard stationed a ·number of intelligence agents in Havana to report on alcohol and alien smuggling networks operating between Havana and the Gulf Coast of the United States. These reports also include valuable inside information on Cuban politics, as well as hundreds of clippings from Havana's daily newspapers. In the postwar years, the United States Federal Bureau of Investigation also maintained a key presence in Cuba, keeping tabs simultaneously on Cuban communists as well as North American organized crime and gambling syndicates operating on the Island. The United States Bureau of Narcotics and Dangerous Drugs took an interest in Cuba in the 1940s and 1950s, particularly in its single-minded pursuit of fugitive gangster Lucky Luciano (who took up residence in Havana following his expulsion from the United States). The U.S. Customs Bureau also kept records relating to violations of the Neutrality Act and weapons smuggling to and from Cuba during the 1950s. The Central Intelligence Agency was also very active in Cuba during the 1940s and 1950s, but very few of their records have been made available to researchers.

Of all these U.S. government sources, the FBI and the Coast Guard maintain by far the most comprehensive and open research materials. Most of the information presented here on criminal syndicates and their relationships with various Cuban political figures in the 1920s has been taken from early Coast Guard Intelligence files. Information on Cuba's political corruption in the 1940s and 1950s comes largely from declassified FBI documents, usually combined with one or more secondary sources. When FBI sources seem to be of dubious reliability, or appear to contradict one another (a common occurrence) I have tried to indicate this ambiguity in the text. It should also be emphasized that by their very nature police records are inherently unreliable. Informants for the FBI were frequently coerced—in some cases the Agency appeared to obtain information by threatening to prosecute certain individuals unless they revealed confidential activities of their peers. In other cases, convicted criminals were offered reduced prison sentences for testifying against others. Needless to say, these tactics do not conform to the conventional social science protocol for eliciting information. They are, however, often the only accounts available that describe the covert dynamics of these vital international events and thus merit consideration.

Note

1. Some recent anthropological, medical anthropological and related works on Cuba that have avoided any discussion of dissident voices include Cole, 1988; Eckstein, 1993; Safa, 1995; Whiteford, 2000; Chomsky, 2001; Waitzkin and Britt, 1989; Feinsilver, 1993; A. Chomsky, 1998; Waitzkin et al., 1997.

6

Imperialism and Health in the Spanish-Cuban-American War, 1897–1902

Cuba's final struggle for independence against Spain began in 1868 with the famous "*Grito de Yara*," a call to arms that mobilized various insurgent groups across Eastern Cuba and eventually inaugurated the unsuccessful Ten Years War (1868–1878). In 1895 the *Grito de Yara* was reinvigorated by the "*Grito de Baire*," a call inspired by the passionate nationalism of Cuba's most eloquent patriot, José Martí. By the 1880s numerous armed bands of Cuban revolutionaries had seized control of rural areas, often working together with sympathetic peasant farmers who provided them with food and other supplies. A powerful exile junta of Cuban nationalists aggressively lobbied for United States support of the Cuban Independence movement in Washington, DC, Philadelphia, New York, and Tampa.

The Spanish response to the increasing power of these Cuban insurgents was severe. In January 1896 General Martinez Campo, who commanded Spain's forces in Cuba, was replaced by General Valeriano Weyler. One of Weyler's first actions (which earned him the nickname "El Carnicero," or "the Butcher") was to institute a brutal policy known as "reconcentration" whereby small farmers were forced to abandon their landholdings, and were herded into cities and towns where they were held in large enclosures similar to concentration camps.

Weyler's reconcentration plan virtually destroyed the economic infrastructure of the island. Commerce declined and food production became seriously diminished. The small farmers incarcerated by Weyler produced almost all of Cuba's foodstuffs, and with their production stopped the island experienced immediate shortages. Before long there was widespread starvation. Food was imported from the United States, but wartime profiteering and import taxes made it largely unaffordable for the poor.

Some observers have claimed that not all of Cuba's wartime misery was caused by the Spanish. One decidedly critical journalist (Rea, 1897) insisted that Cuban insurgents themselves maintained a policy of destroying any rural farms that denied them support, and burned farms and sugar mills of those suspected of loyalty to Spain. The subsequent agricultural devastation was then blamed on the Spanish to generate additional sympathy for the rebel cause from North American journalists (particularly those of the Hearst newspaper chain).

Even if the Cuban rebels were themselves partially responsible for some of the destruction of agricultural production in the countryside[1], the Spanish reconcentration policy alone was enough to bring about serious health problems to the island. The disruption of food production along with the forced relocation of large numbers of rural dwellers into crowded townships provided a perfect environment for the spread of infectious disease. The camps were provided with few amenities, and the combination of hunger, crowding and lack of clean water or waste removal led to severe outbreaks of gastrointestinal diseases, as well as crowd diseases such as measles, smallpox, plague, and tuberculosis. The *reconcentrados* also had few defenses against mosquitoes, and epidemics of yellow fever and malaria followed as well. In 1896 one North American congressman traveled to Cuba and reported finding, "Four hundred women and children lying on the stone floors [in an abandoned hospital] in an indescribably horrible state of emaciation and disease" (Bonsal, 1896).

Disease outbreaks were not limited to individual townships. Illness, malnutrition and infection flowed rapidly from the rural *reconcentrados* into the urban centers and a number of epidemics followed. Each successive wave of disease further weakened the population and created more social upheaval in its wake. By 1897 the urban infrastructure (food distribution, street cleaning, sanitation) of Havana had virtually collapsed and mortality rates were skyrocketing. In the words of one historian (Stephen, 1977), "The total loss to Cuba's population as a result of [the Spanish policy of] reconcentration was probably 400,000—possibly the highest death rate per capita of any war of independence." Over 100,00 small farms, 3,000 livestock ranches, 800 tobacco and 700 coffee farms were destroyed during the war, and sugar production dropped from one million tons in 1894, down to as low as 225,000 in 1896 (Perez, 1983).

Concerned about reports of Havana's deteriorating health profile, as well as the possibility of epidemic disease spreading from Cuba to southern port cities in the United States through steamship traffic, the United States Public Health Service (then under the control of the U.S. Marine Hospital Service, abbreviated as USPHS) sent a representative named W.F. Brunner to Cuba in 1897 to monitor conditions and assist in the inspection of ships bound for U.S. ports. Sanitary Commissioner Brunner also compiled weekly reports of deaths from infectious disease compiled from mortuary data, and provided a number of detailed (and relatively impartial) eyewitness descriptions of health conditions in Cuba during this time.

In his first dispatch from Havana, Brunner noted that in the month of April 1897 alone there were a total of 1,062 deaths reported in Havana (which at the time, had a total population of only about 230,000 inhabitants[2]). Of these deaths, approximately 600 were caused by infectious diseases. These were further broken down as follows : eighty-two deaths from diseases caused by insect vectors (such as malaria and yellow fever), 317 deaths from diseases caused by respiratory borne infections (such as tuberculosis or smallpox) and 196 deaths from waterborne diseases such as enteritis and dysentery.

Health conditions continued to deteriorate through the summer months. In his health report for the month of August, Brunner describes in detail the wretched condition of the city and its inhabitants,

> In spite of the heavy rains which deluge the streets, running over the sidewalks in many places, the city appears to contain more filth than ever: human excrement is to be found on the sidewalks, offensive odors assail the nostrils and it is impossible to properly describe the absolute want of sanitary measures, the absolute disregard of health laws. The waters of the bay are reeking with the filth poured into it from the city and every vessel leaving here for the U.S. should be regarded with suspicion. . . . I am more convinced than ever that this city is a constant menace to the health of the United States and will remain so until modern medical science shall be employed to remedy the evils that have existed here for nearly two centuries (Brunner to USPHS, August 4, 1897).

The ongoing arrival of new Spanish soldiers also meant there was a critical mass of immigrants on the island who had no previous exposure or immunity to yellow fever. Many of these Spaniards quickly fell ill and were placed in military hospitals. This practice served to amplify the yellow fever outbreak into a major epidemic. Crowded conditions in the military hospitals made it impossible to isolate or quarantine yellow fever patients, and as a result, soldiers who were hospitalized for any reason often came down with yellow fever while in the hospital. Smallpox, known in Europe for many generations, correspondingly did not appear to affect the Spanish soldiers as severely as the Cubans.

In the late 1800s, the city of Havana took part of its drinking water from the Almendares River, which flowed virtually unfiltered into the city's spring-fed reservoir. During summer months increasing rains washed more and more of Havana's refuse into the river, and thus into the city's drinking water supply. Severe outbreaks of waterborne diseases were reported, which further weakened the urban population. The following table (compiled by Brunner) shows the increase in deaths from diarrheal diseases for Havana alone during the summer of 1897:

Table 6.1
Increase in Havana's mortality rates during the war against Spain,
summer 1897

Month	deaths from diarrheal diseases	death from all causes	annual ratio per 1000
April	64	1062	63.32
May	126	1015	60.9
June	143	1041	62.46
July	171	1193	71.52
August	291	1439	86.34
September	411	1778	106.68

As a result of these deteriorating health conditions, the mortality rate in Havana continued to rise. In September of 1897 it climbed to 106.68 deaths per 1,000 inhabitants—an astronomically high figure. For the sake of comparison, the mortality rates in New Orleans (a city with similar climate and ecological conditions) was only twenty-eight per 1,000 in the late 1800s, and Milwaukee's rate (a northern city with fewer infectious conditions) was only 18.5 per 1,000 (Leavitt, 1983). Unfortunately USPHS Commissioner Brunner did not report on health conditions outside of the capital city, but other observers recorded equally terrible figures for the remainder of the island. In Santiago, for instance, one observer estimated the overall mortality rate in 1898 to be around eighty-two per 1,000 (Porter, 1899).

In addition to the contaminated water, Brunner also described Cuba's impoverished urban population as surviving on marginal or spoiled foodstuffs. The resulting diarrhea and malnutrition subsequently made them more vulnerable to the infectious diseases circulating in the cities. By the fall of 1897, the first cases of deaths due to starvation were noted in Havana. In his October report, Brunner describes the increasing sickness and desperation of the urban poor,

> There are fourteen deaths [in the week of October 4, 1897] attributed to starvation which is what I would estimate to be about one third the actual number of deaths from that cause and the next few weeks will show a more distressing condition of affairs. Just opposite to the office of the [public health] Service a wholesale grocery firm gives away a portion of rice to all who apply for it twice a week. Hundreds of thin emaciated people drag themselves there to partake of the bounty and it is a gruesome sight to observe the condition or rather lack of physical condition of the crowd.

Conditions continued to deteriorate through the winter months. Brunner's report from November, 1897 describes an epidemic of typhoid fever in Matanzas "with an enormous death rate," as well as intensification of the smallpox epidemic and ongoing mortality from intestinal diseases. Havana and the interior towns remained virtually without any health or sanitation measures to stop the spread of these diseases.

The U.S. Presence

In the spring of 1898 the United States actively entered into the war against Spain on the side of the Cuban nationalists. These actions were precipitated by a number of factors. Journalists from Hearst newspapers had been sending vivid, heart-rending dispatches to New York detailing the misery and suffering of the *reconcentrados*, a practice that generated tremendous public outrage against Spain in the United States. At the same time the Cuban revolutionary junta in exile greatly increased its lobbying efforts with the newly inaugurated McKinley administration, as well as with a number of North American businesses. Many U.S. businessmen appear to have been promised lucrative concessions by Cuban lobbyists if they would use their influence with the McKinley administration to advance the Cuban cause.[3] U.S. senator Redfield Proctor was especially influential in lobbying the American business community to support intervention in Cuba.

In the early spring of 1898 two key events effectively propelled the United States into the Cuban War of Independence. On February 9, the *New York Journal* published a secret letter, allegedly intercepted by the Cubans, from Spain's ambassador to the United States that derided and criticized the McKinley administration. This letter was viewed as highly disrespectful and greatly inflamed public opinion against Spain. Six days later, the *U.S.S. Maine* exploded in Havana harbor.

The question of how the U.S.S. Maine blew up has still not been definitively answered. At the time, the Hearst newspapers insisted the ship was blown up by a Spanish mine in an act of deliberate aggression against the United States. The present Cuban government, on the other hand, has always maintained that the United States deliberately exploded the ship in order to have a pretext to invade Cuba and thwart Cuban independence[4] (detailed in the *New York Times*, June 8, 1960). A less politicized (and probably more accurate) version holds that the ship blew up by accident when coal stores spontaneously combusted, igniting a nearby store of gunpowder.

In any event, collective North American outrage at what was perceived as Spanish brutality and treachery, combined with an increasing awareness of the commercial possibilities available in Cuba, plus worries that the island might fall into the hands of a hostile European power, were sufficient to compel the United States to enter the War. On April 19, 1898 the United States Congress voted 311 to 6 (in the House) and 42 to 35 (in the Senate) in favor of a Joint Resolution for war with Spain. Included in this Resolution was the Teller Amendment (sponsored by Senator Henry Moore Teller of Colorado) that disclaimed any American intention to colonize Cuba, and promised a swift military exit once the island was pacified.[5]

The actual fighting of the Spanish-Cuban-American War was relatively short. By late in the summer of 1898, Spanish forces had been defeated in the Philippine Islands and in Santiago, Cuba. By December a peace accord was reached. In this agreement, Spain ceded the Philippines, Puerto Rico and Guam to the United States for U.S. $20 million, and renounced all rights to Cuba, which was declared independent. By January, Spanish forces were evacuated from Cuba and the island was placed under the control of the United States military.

Health and the Politics of Annexation

One of the most immediate concerns of the U.S. military upon the cessation of the war was the terrible health and sanitation conditions of Cuba's cities. Havana's epidemics were considered a grave health risk to U.S. soldiers and a potential menace to the southern port cities of New Orleans and Tampa. One North American observer, in fact, argued that Cuba should be annexed to the United States as a means of controlling the spread of yellow fever and other infectious diseases,

> And we need [to annex] Cuba for self-preservation, from the sanitary point of view. Everybody knows what an awful scourge yellow fever has been to us, especially in our southern ports. The plague has been traced to Cuba almost every time it has appeared among us. Bad sanitary conditions, filth of all kinds, utter disregard for all regulations that conduce to public health—these have remained for hundreds of years and will continue unless we take hold and clean up . . . and keep the island clean (Hyatt and Hyatt, 1898:2).

Health, of course, was not the only reason North American observers argued for annexation. Cuba was also considered extremely strategic from a military point of view, and to be quite economically valuable to U.S. business interests. In addition to their plea for annexation of Cuba on health grounds, Hyatt and Hyatt are also careful to note " . . . in Cuba there is for the businessman a future beyond the dreams of avarice" (1898:iv).

The question of Cuban annexation following the Spanish-Cuban-American War was quite controversial in the United States. A number of leading U.S. citizens strongly opposed both the entry of the U.S. into the Cuban conflict and the possible annexation of Cuba that might result. In the late 1800s these individuals formed an Anti-Imperialist league to lobby against U.S. involvement in Cuba. The league included such prominent leaders as former U.S. Presidents Cleveland and Harrison, along with notable capitalists like Andrew Carnegie and literary figures such as Mark Twain.

Interesting enough, it was the annexationists rather than the anti-imperialists who were most successful at cooping a rhetoric of compassionate humanitarianism to justify their cause, as is evident in the following passage (taken from Porter, 1898:6),

> Whatever form the government of Cuba may take, the responsibility of the commercial and industrial rehabilitation of the island must rest with the U.S. The power that forced the Spanish to evacuate the island is the power that the world will hold responsible for the future welfare of its people. . . . For the U.S. to desert Cuba in its hour of need would be more inhuman than it would have been to have left it to Weyler and his policy of extermination.

Other North Americans argued in favor of U.S. imperialism in the Caribbean, invoking paternalistic (and racist) metaphors of "progress," "destiny," and "civilization" to justify increasing North American control (see Clark, 1898:xvi).

Conservatives, on the other hand, argued against formal annexation of Cuba on racial and cultural grounds. From their point of view, annexation would have meant granting U.S. citizenship to large numbers of Afro-Cubans, including many recently freed slaves. The racial segregation policies in place in the United States at this time made annexation deeply unpopular among white southerners. Even "white" Cubans were viewed with some suspicion by conservative Anglo-Americans, and were frequently described as members of a lesser Hispanic race with an innately unstable temperament that made them less qualified for membership in the "civilized" United States.[6]

It is also important to note that many Cubans, as well as Spaniards living in Cuba, were themselves in favor of annexation to the United States at this time. After the cessation of hostilities against Spain, Cuba's various military leaders quickly split off into highly personalistic factions, each with its own cadre of armed followers. By 1900 two distinct political parties had formed along these lines: 1) the Cuban National Party, made up primarily of supporters of General Maximo Gómez; 2) the Republican Party, made up of "those who had split from General Gómez and become his enemies" (Norton, 1900: 174). The fear of many Cubans was that without the stabilizing force of the United States army in place, these two political parties would begin fighting with one another to gain sole control of the newly independent Cuban republic, and a protracted civil war would result. For a nation still reeling from the destruction, disease, and violence of years of warfare against Spain, annexation seemed to promise peace and economic recovery. As Matthews (1899:42) noted,

> Every person of the Pro-Spanish class, those who sympathized with Spain and hoped she would defeat the revolutionists, wanted the U.S. to retain control of the island. . . . The merchants of the island, almost without exception, wanted American control, because only in that way did they see any assurance of stability in commerce, and any hope of the full development of the business possibilities of the island. The peasants and laborers . . . long only for peace.

The purpose of this digression into attitudes about annexation is to illustrate that there was no single overriding commercial motive in the United States' decision to intervene in Cuba, and certainly no universal consensus within the United States (or Cuba) regarding annexation. The entry of the United States into Cuba's war against Spain was not (as recent newspaper articles in Cuba have claimed), "an annexationist war against Cuban independence." Instead, the situation was much more complex and nuanced. Many of the major North American decision-makers at the time appeared to have highly disparate and incompatible agendas.

For some North Americans, the U.S. military presence in Cuba was viewed primarily as a humanitarian mission intended to relieve the overwhelming suffering, misery and disease suffered by Havana's urban poor and the rural *reconcentrados* during the War. For others, U.S. control of Cuba was viewed as opening a vast new horizon of commercial possibilities—a chance for American business to seize control of lucrative resources that had previously lain stagnant under Spain's stifling mercantilism. And for other North Americans, the Cuba question was primarily one of national defense interests for the United States. As Porter (1899:38) stated, "To the United States as a military nation and naval power, Cuba is a necessity; without Cuba you have simply Key West. . . . Having this naval defense, which makes the U.S. non-attackable from Cape Hatteras to the Rio Grande, with how much more efficacy, and without danger, you can move your armies."

In these various annexation arguments it is possible to find extreme liberals who rejected annexation on the basis of anti-imperialism, siding with extreme conservatives who rejected annexation on the grounds of racism and ethnic bias. Moderates maintained various intermediate positions. Typically there was consensus that the United States had some obligation to "stabilize" Cuba, and to help it recover from the political and economic devastation brought on by years of warfare. But how this obligation might be met (prolonged military occupation, establishing a political protectorate, expanding commercial ties or outright annexation) was never satisfactorily agreed upon.

Imperial Health and Sanitation

Given the ambivalence in Washington, DC about the overall goal of U.S. military occupation of Cuba, the army was uncertain how to interpret its role at the end of the war. Was it intended to prepare Cuba for annexation to the United States? To stabilize the country politically and depart as soon as possible, leaving Cuba to determine its own fate as an independent republic? Or to facilitate the expansion of North American capitalist enterprise on the island? Groups within the United States government seemed equally divided regarding these contradictory goals, leaving the occupation forces without a clear mission or departure strategy. With its larger purpose in Cuba undecided, the U.S. army focused its energies on immediately attainable and politically favorable goals of improving Cuba's health and sanitation infrastructure.

The urgency of these tasks was quite apparent. By the end of the war sanitary conditions in Havana had deteriorated to the point where many U.S. troops refused to occupy the government buildings vacated by the Spanish. "Havana is viler than words can express," wrote one visiting journalist at the close of the war (Porter, 1899). The departure of the Spanish exacerbated these conditions further. General Brooke, the commander in chief of the U.S. occupation forces, himself described postwar Havana as follows,

> The physical condition of the city could only be described as frightful. There were several thousands *reconcentrados* in and about, who had been herding like swine and perishing like flies. They were found dead in the streets and in their noisome quarters, where disease and starvation were rampant. Other thousands were lacking in food, clothing and medicine. The regular service of the city was practically paralyzed—street cleaning at best a farce, suspended and the houses of assistance and hospitals destitute of resources, even food. No sanitary measures or rules were in force,

and the thronging population—soldiers, *reconcentrados*, natives and citizens—used the streets or any open place for deposit of refuse and filth of all kinds. A woman, killed by a railway train, lay on a principal street for eight hours because an ambulance and the proper officials could not be found to remove her. It was nearly the same with all other branches of the city administration. Officials, clerks and employees had been unpaid for many months, and the public offices were practically abandoned (Brooke, 1899:7).

General Brooke soon put the U.S. army to work. Between January and November of 1899, 5.5 million rations of food were distributed to the Cuban people by the U.S. army, and *reconcentrados* were allowed to reclaim their land and plant new crops (Langley, 1989). A smallpox vaccination campaign was instigated and an aggressive street-cleaning program was instituted in all the major cities. The Marine Hospital Service (inspired by the theories of Cuban physician Carlos Finlay) also began successfully experimenting with mosquito control as a means to combat yellow fever. In urban areas American soldiers were organized into sanitary brigades that conducted a house-by-house health census to determine which dwellings were most in need of assistance. Refuse was removed, waterworks repaired, sewers constructed, swamps filled in, wharves built, jails renovated and major engineering works undertaken (Bangs, 1902; Brooke, 1899; Matthews, 1899; Porter, 1899).

According to one source (*New York Times*, March 18, 1901), over 55,075 tons of street dirt were removed from Havana alone. Over forty-seven percent of Havana's macadam streets were repaved during the occupation, and many dirt paths paved for the first time. In Santiago, ten miles of new asphalt streets were laid, "sewer flats" were dredged, a sea wall constructed, and new water and sewer lines were laid throughout the city (Brooke, 1899). These improvements were described by the *New York Times* (March 18, 1901) as follows:

> The water supply of the city [Havana] is now in the hands of a modern water department. We wish the same could be said of New York. The mains and services required a good deal of attention and had to be generally overhauled. The leakage was heavy and the house waste much in excess of the useful employment of water for all purposes. This has been largely corrected . . . A house-to-house inspection has been made, resulting in important reforms in the sanitary condition of dwellings and in checking water waste. . . . This is practical sanitation of the very best kind . . .

Furthermore, thanks to Carlos Finlay's discoveries, a mosquito control program was instituted that reduced yellow fever mortality in Havana from a colonial average of 706 deaths per year (recorded from 1870–1900) down to only eighteen deaths in 1901 (Danielson, 1979). This was accomplished not by improvements in clinical medicine or treatment for yellow fever, but by "direct destruction of the insect" followed by a program of "destroying its breeding places . . . and by draining low lands by ditching" (Bangs, 1902:325). A house-to-house inspection campaign was organized that destroyed an estimated 90 percent of domestic mosquito larvae (Bangs, 1902).

Sanitary Commissioner Brunner described immediate results from these programs. In March of 1899 he wrote to the USPHS, "In all probability the death rate during this week has been the lowest recorded since 1894. There have been but 187 deaths during this time, from all causes. No deaths are reported either from yellow fever or smallpox." In May, he stated, "Beyond diphtheria and measles and the usual death rate from TB there is but little to mention as to epidemic diseases."

The cumulative results of these various health and sanitation improvements were striking. In only five years, overall mortality in Havana plunged dramatically from approximately ninety-one per 1,000 to 22.1 per 1,000. Typhoid mortality dropped from an all-time high of 650 per 100,00 in Havana in 1898 to around fifty per 100,000 in 1903 and tuberculosis deaths declined sharply from 117.25 per 10,000 in 1898 to 37.71 per 10,000 in 1903 (Finlay Institute, 1925; LeRoy y Cassa, 1922).

The army's public works program was not limited to health and sanitation. During the occupation U.S. troops also modernized the urban infrastructure of Havana, constructed the Malecón (Havana's famous seaside promenade), inaugurated a public school system, collected taxes and established Cuba's first national treasury, reorganized the University of Havana, reformed the prison system, introduced judicial reform (and habeas corpus), regulated the British-owned railway system and organized municipal governments (Jenks, 1928).

At the time of the occupation, the U.S. army's achievements were considered by many Cubans and Americans to be nothing short of miraculous. "The dullest clod," wrote one enthused American visitor, "would come back [from occupied Cuba] with impressions the proper presentation of which to the great American public would inspire in the latter a pride so great it could hardly be adequately described" (Bangs, 1902:340). Many leading Cuban physicians echoed these sentiments, praising the health accomplishments of Carlos Finlay and the American army in eradicating yellow fever, and later referring to this period as the "golden era of sanitation" in Cuba (Barnet, 1905; Exposito, 1947; Hard, 1928; Lindsay, 1911; LeRoy y Cassa, 1921; 1922; Lopez del Valle, 1924).

Despite winning many official words of praise for their health achievements, these military programs were not without controversy. Sanitary commissioner Brunner himself criticized the U.S. military authorities for taking sole credit for Cuba's abrupt mortality shift, and insisted a good deal of the decline in infectious disease should in actuality be understood as a natural phenomenon resulting from the elimination of susceptible individuals from the population during the war years. In July, 1899 Brunner detailed these reflections in a lengthy report on the various social and environmental factors involved in configuring Cuba's abrupt postwar mortality decline. Brunner's astute analysis is worth quoting at length for its insights into Havana's abrupt mortality shift,

> In view of the frequent comparisons of the present and past sanitary condition of Havana . . . it would seem to be interesting to mention some factors which must be considered in making such a comparison intelligently. . . . The years from 1895 to 1898 were the years of war. In 1897 and 1898 the city passed through a period of extreme suffering; insufficient and improper food for very many and starvation for a large number; neglect of medical care for the sick and insufficient and improper hospital accommodation etc.

> The effect of these conditions . . . on the present death rate is from two factors: 1) a number of people are left in a weakened condition and are less able to resist ordinary diseases; 2) a large proportion of the old people; those suffering from chronic maladies; and those whose vitality was less than normal, died during this period. The survivors being those of greater than average natural vitality, or better physical surroundings. The first factor tends to raise the present death rate; the latter to lower it. . . . It would seem then, that the resultant of the two factors above mentioned would be to lessen the death rate now, and to give us a lower rate for some time to come. If, in addition to this, we consider the appalling mortality of young children during the two years mentioned, and the lessened birth rate during the same period, this conclusion will be strengthened. Very few

young children were left in a weakened condition—they died! The same is true of old people. In Havana I have no knowledge to be depended upon for the birth rate during the period mentioned. But in Matanzas the statistics collected by General Wilson show that in 1898 the births in that city almost ceased, and were, I am informed, confined to the wealthier classes.

Now children under five years of age furnish, normally much more than their proportion of mortality (most during the two or three years) as of course, do old people; and the marked diminution, almost extinction of these classes, must tend also to lessen the mortality now, and in the immediate future.

Acting entirely on the same lines is the after effect of the great epidemics of smallpox and yellow fever prevailing all over the Island in 1895 and 1897. This influence is especially felt in lessening the death rate from these diseases; but also affects the death rate from other diseases by the number of those of deficient vitality that perish. As is well known, smallpox is especially deadly in the very young and very old . . .

It is fair to predict then, that the conditions which prevailed from 1896–1898 will tend to lower our death rate for some time to come; say a year and a half or two years and a half, from the evacuation, its influence gradually lessening to zero.

The better care of the indigent classes; issuing of rations; care of the sick in hospitals and at dispensaries; issuing medicine; and the whole system of public assistance in fact (which is unquestionably well administered) also lowers the bills of mortality below the normal of former years. The sanitary measures adopted since the American occupation also act in the same direction, lessening the death rate. The effect of this factor will be permanent and increasing (Brunner to USPHS, July 24, 1899).

Brunner's observations on the nature of Havana's mortality changes were not well received by his superiors in Washington, DC.[7] Shortly after this critical report was circulated, Brunner was charged with attempting to discredit the health and sanitation work of the U.S. army and was dismissed from his position as USPHS sanitary commissioner by military officials. Brunner subsequently found employment in the health department in Savannah, Georgia, and one of his assistants was promoted to take his place in Havana. As might be expected, subsequent USPHS reports from Havana to Washington, DC lack Brunner's critical perspective and social commentary, and consist of little more than rote recitation of local health statistics.

Other observers also found reason to criticize the U.S. army's aggressive sanitation programs in Cuba. In many cases, these public health efforts were undertaken with no regard for local customs and with no respect for individual rights or personal privacy. Violent enforcement of health codes was not uncommon. The army's repressive practices were described by one observer as follows:

> The resistance on the part of the native population [to compliance with sanitation orders] was even more stubborn than that of the Spanish soldiers to our forces around Santiago. The doors of houses had to be smashed in, people making sewers of the thoroughfares were publicly horsewhipped in the streets of Santiago; eminently respectable citizens were forcibly brought before the commanding general and sentenced to aid in cleaning the streets they were in the habit of defiling. The campaign has ended in the complete surrender to the sanitary authorities, and the inhabitants of Santiago, regardless of class, have had their first object lesson in the new order of things inaugurated by the war (Porter, 1899:63).

Furthermore, these draconian policies were often imposed with an explicitly racist rhetoric that caricatured Cubans as recalcitrant, uncivilized children incapable of tending to basic matters of hygiene or sanitation for themselves. The *New York Times* stated as much with an editorial that read in part, (March 18, 1901, p. 6),

> To originate a scheme of public sanitation is something for which the Spanish-American is constitutionally and temperamentally unfitted. Whether he is able to carry on a work of this kind already begun . . . would seem to depend a good deal upon the extent to which he is willing to entrust its execution to those whose judgment in such matters is better than his own.

Needless to say, these imperial attitudes and activities on the part of U.S. officials created resentment among the Cubans. Despite the numerous physical improvements in Havana and other cities, pressure began building for the U.S. occupation to come to a close. After decades of fighting for independence against Spain, Cubans were unwilling to surrender to the imperial rule of the United States.

The End of the Occupation

Many Cuban nationalists were justifiably angered by the imposition of American military rule in Cuba following the end of Spanish colonial rule. While some individuals in the U.S. government were sympathetic to the cause of *Cuba Libre,* others continued to lobby for the U.S. annexation of Cuba. Many of those who sympathized with the Cuban nationalists, however, also voiced persistent doubts about Cuba's ability to govern itself in ways that were compatible with American interests (including health interests) in the region. The result was an uncomfortable compromise in which American troops were withdrawn after three years (to placate Cuban nationalists), but on the condition that Cuba continue to submit a certain degree of paternalistic American supervision of its affairs (to placate the annexationists). The logic of this compromise was described in a letter from General Leonard Wood (in charge of U.S. forces in Havana) written in 1902,

> We have spent enormous sums of money and thousands of valuable lives in bringing Cuba up to her present condition. If we allow her to go to smash, we have got to do it all over again whether we want to or not, because we cannot permit the internal conditions to recur which existed at the time of our intervention. In short, every motive of public policy and common sense and self-interest points to a liberal and wise treatment of Cuba. It is more important, in fact, to us than to her (Letter from Wood to Henry Allen White, July 14, 1902).

Particularly worrisome for many American statesmen and businessmen was the extent to which Cuba's indigenous political groups remained violently factionalized during the American occupation. Shortly before the withdrawal of U.S. troops, one American soldier stated, "[I]f we [the U.S. Army] should go home, our transport would be lighted out of the harbor . . . by the flames of anarchy; but that is none of our business" (quoted in Matthews, 1899:41). Enough powerful Americans, however, apparently did feel believe that Cuban politics should become "our business" that they conditioned the withdrawal of U.S. troops upon the Cuban congress' acceptance of the Platt Amendment as an article of the new constitution.

This amendment was proposed by Senator Orville Platt ostensibly as a means to prevent instability in the new republic by allowing the United States government to intervene in Cuba should an "economic or political crisis" occur. Senator Platt was once quoted as stating that, "the United States cannot be satisfied with the ordinary South American republic in Cuba, which was one of revolution, turmoil and a confiscator of debts" (quoted in Turner, 1932). Platt argued that United States supervision in Cuba would "insist upon a quiet, orderly and peaceful government there . . . which would insure our peace and quiet and safeguard our interest . . . " (quoted in Turner, 1932).

The Platt amendment has frequently been criticized by contemporary historians as a tool of U.S. imperial domination of Cuba's political affairs (Benjamin, 1974; Benjamin, 1990; Perez, 1986; Perez, 1988; Simons, 1996). In some regards this critical interpretation of the Platt Amendment is correct, but closer examination of Cuban history reveals that this imperial domination was often ambiguously deployed, depending on the goals of the particular U.S. administration in power. For some American statesmen, supervision of Cuba's affairs was a guise to facilitate capitalist penetration of Cuba, but for others (particularly Elihu Root, Rooseveldt's Secretary of State) it allegedly represented (in the words of one critical scholar) "an honest attempt at state-building," (Jenks, 1928:85).

At the urging of these more altruistic voices, and to try and deflect charges that the Platt Amendment was an intended as a tool of U.S. imperial expansion, Congress also passed the Teller Amendment. This article was designed to protect Cuba from any overzealous interpretation of the Platt Amendment on the part of American capitalists. The text of the Teller Amendment read as follows:

> The United States hereby disclaims any disposition, or intention to exercise sovereignty, jurisdiction or control over the said Island, except for the pacification thereof, and asserts its determination, when that is accomplished, to leave the government and control of the Island to its people.

In terms of health and sanitation, the Platt Amendment is significant in that (in addition to four general articles specifying the conditions under which the American government would intervene in Cuba), a fifth article was added that was designed to force the Cuban government to maintain the health and sanitation programs initiated under the U.S. military occupation. This article allowed for further American intervention if the Cubans failed to maintain acceptable levels of health and sanitation. The text of article five read as follows:

That the government of Cuba will execute, and as far as necessary extend, the plans already devised or other plans to be mutually agreed upon, for the sanitation of the cities of the island, to the end that a recurrence of epidemic and infectious diseases may be prevented, thereby assuring protection to the people and commerce of Cuba, as well as the southern ports of the U.S. and the people residing therein.

The imposition of article five of the Platt Amendment resulted in an intense politicization of health on the island throughout the Platt Era. Any Cuban leader who appeared to be negligent of public health could be accused by his rivals of endangering Cuba's fragile sovereignty by facilitating another U.S. military occupation. From 1902 until the abrogation of the Platt Amendment in 1933, health propaganda figured prominently in Cuba's internal political disputes.

Notes

1. For further discussion of the role of Cuban forces in contributing to the devastation of the country, see Pratt, 1950.
2. This figure is taken from Norton, 1926.
3. One of these individuals was Horatio Rubens. Rubens began his career as a clerk in Elihu Root's law firm, and later became an ardent champion of the Cuban cause. He used his political connections via Root to lobby U.S. congressmen on behalf of the Cubans and personally outfitted over seventeen expeditions to Cuba. In the late 1800s Rubens created and financed a number of Cuban propaganda bureaus in the United States. After the War, Rubens was rewarded by the new Cuban regime with lucrative railway concessions and eventually he became president of the Cuban Railroad Corporation. At one point Rubens allegedly told one U.S. investor in Cuba that he (Rubens) "had sufficient influence with the Cuban Government to obtain anything he desired from it" (quoted in affidavit of Woolsey H. Field re Rubens Property and Revolution Proposition, September 20, 1907).
4. In 1960 the Castro regime changed all of Cuba's elementary school textbooks regarding the Maine incident. These changes were detailed in a New York Times article which stated, "All history books are being changed [in Cuba] to conform with the attitude of Dr. Castro's officials, who have repeatedly declared the United States is 'Cuba's greatest enemy' (*New York Times*, June 8, 1960).
5. For a more detailed chronology of these events, see (http://www.loc.gov/rr/hispanic/1898/chronology.html)
6. It is worth noting that from day one race and racism were fundamental elements of "the Cuba question" in both the liberal and conservative positions in the United States. "Liberals" at the time believed in racial hierarchies, but felt that "the lesser races" were capable of learning or acquiring civilization under the benevolent leadership of the more advanced races. Colonialism was thus justified with hu-

manitarian rhetoric. "Conservatives" on the other hand, tended toward more bio-logical determinism and did not believe the so-called lesser races were capable of acquiring "civilization." As a result, conservatives tended toward strict segregation.

7. Brunner had previously antagonized the army command when he wrote in an earlier report that he had personally taken control of a hospital sanitation program, and that his efforts were "without question the only instance of intelligent and efficient disinfection ever practiced in a building in the city of Havana." To make matters worse, this report was quoted in a Havana newspaper.

7

Caudillismo, Imperialism and Health, 1902–1909

The conflicting agendas manifest between United States government, military and business interests in Cuba were mirrored by similar conflicts between different Cuban political factions themselves. Just as a wide array of motives (economic, strategic, political, humanitarian) could be attributed to various United States interests, indigenous Cuban leaders also expressed conflicting goals and plans for the newly liberated republic. Some Cuban revolutionaries clearly sought independence from Spain for reasons of patriotism and humanitarian anticolonialism. Others, however, appeared to be motivated largely by financial goals—specifically the economic opportunities (i.e., graft, corruption, sinecures, and access to the wealth of the national treasury) afforded by political office in an independent republic.

Attributing economic motivation to Cuban revolutionaries is very much at odds with contemporary scholarship in Latin American Studies. Most sources portray Cuba's independence fighters as motivated solely by ideals of national sovereignty and anti-colonialism. In this conventional historical narrative, United States interventions in Cuba following the Spanish-Cuban-American War served to rob these patriots of a truly independent republic, forcibly subjecting them to "neocolonial exploitation" until the socialist revolution in 1959. This version of history is frequently used to rationalize the powerful anti-Americanism of the Castro regime.

A number of observers (both Cuban and American) in the early 1900s, however, described economic rather than altruistic motives for many key individuals in the independence movement.[1] In 1899 one

North American journalist reported a conversation with a member of the Cuban military assembly who stated quite openly, "We are willing to give the United States complete control of every kind, except political annexation. You may annex us commercially—that is what we want; but we also want independence—in name at least." To this the reporter replied, "In other words, you want the offices and the opportunities of office?" The military leader affirmed that was indeed the case (Reported in Matthews, 1899:41). Irene Wright offered a similarly forthright analysis in her report from Havana in 1910,

> Americans, when they rushed to the aid of Free Cuba in 1898, supposed that they were intervening on behalf of an oppressed people struggling for justice. The truth is, they championed a horde of disgruntled political aspirants after "jobs" who cloaked their real aims in the mantles of not a few visionaries working with them, inspired, unquestionably by genuine patriotism. . . . These two very different varieties of "patriots," the one class working to their own personal ends and the other to accomplish an "ideal" found their joint efforts against Spain seconded in the provinces by the simple countryman . . . [who] desired solely peace and a good market for his crops (1910:167).

Of the two groups of Cuban "patriots" described by Wright, it was unfortunately the avaricious office-seekers rather than the "genuine visionaries" who had the most lasting (and destructive) impact in shaping the political character of postwar Cuba. As Aguilar (1972:28) has stated, "The enlightened patriciate had been decimated in the fight for independence, and the opportunists, newcomers and speculators who replaced them, without any trace of patriotism, had taken advantage of American penetration and become interested defenders of the status quo." The entire Platt era, in fact, was characterized by continual cycles of violence and instability as rival factions of office-seekers, previously united in the struggle against Spain, fought one another for access to the spoils of war—government jobs in the new republic. The following chapter will detail the nature of Cuban politics during this era, and discuss the impact of this political factionalism, violence and instability on patterns of health and disease.

Caudillismo and the Roots of Instability

The "disgruntled political aspirants" who came to dominate Cuban politics in the Platt era exemplified the Latin American political tradition of *caudillismo*. The term *caudillo* literally means "man on horse-back" and refers to traditional Latin strongman authoritarian rule. Nearly every country in Latin America has had a *caudillo* period when political power was seized by force and government viewed as a spoils system for the victors (Wolf and Hansen, 1966). Most often this period followed the collapse of Spanish colonialism, when the resulting power vacuum left a country vulnerable to takeover by ambitious leaders who sought to enrich themselves and their followers by plundering the national treasury. Eric Wolf and Edward Hansen have described *caudillo* government as defined by four essential characteristics:

1. The repeated emergence of armed patron-client sets, cemented by personal ties of dominance and submission, and by a common desire to obtain wealth by force of arms;
2. The lack of institutionalized means for succession to offices;
3. The use of violence in political competition;
4. The repeated failures of incumbent leaders to guarantee their tenures as chieftains (Wolf and Hansen, 1966:169).

One researcher has described the configuration of politics and economics that characterizes *caudillo* rule as a form of "political capitalism" (Scott, 1972). Political capitalism usually involves the appearance of a free market economy, but in reality economic exchange or accumulation of capital nearly always involves a significant political dimension. Many markets are not, in fact, free but are deliberately controlled and manipulated to enhance the power of the leader in ways that may not be readily apparent to an outside observer. In the words of Scott (1972:52),

Politically oriented capitalism, whatever particular form it takes, involves the granting by the state of privileged opportunities for profit. Such openings are available only to those with connections or to those who can pay for influence. The "capitalists" in these circumstances are often officials inasmuch as state administrators are best placed to take advantage of the opportunities.

Caudillos employ political capitalism to establish and maintain lucrative economic monopolies for themselves in both the informal and formal economies. Indeed, history reveals that in many cases of strongman rule in Latin America, the entire governing body and the national economy have come under the personal control of the leader and dedicated to enhancing his personal wealth, status and power. "Government" of this type has been described in many parts of Latin America and the Caribbean during the twentieth century, including Nicaragua under Somoza (Chevalier, 1965; Guillermoprieto, 1994), the Dominican Republic under Trujillo (Goff and Locker, 1969; Galíndez, 1965), Venezuela in the "*caudillo* years" of the early twentieth century (Wolf and Hansen, 1972), and Haiti under Duvalier (Scott, 1972; Trouillot, 1990).

Rafael Trujillo, for instance, followed a typical *caudillo* pattern during his rule in the Dominican Republic, using his political power to control many economic activities in both the formal and informal sectors of the economy for his own benefit. One critic described these practices as follows,

> Trujillo . . . saw in the entire economic process a source of dominion as potent as the army, as strong as the most rigid political structure. Funds collected from the public and from illicit operations were invested in every conceivable agricultural and industrial enterprise; monopolies usually followed. Import-export taxes and license fees facilitated the harassment and eventual takeover of corporations dealing in foreign trade, the lifeblood of the economy. . . . It has been estimated that between 65 and 85 percent of the entire economy eventually ended up in his hands (Goff and Locker, 1969:279).

The emergence of *caudillismo* and instability following the end of Spanish rule in Latin America followed as a logical outgrowth of the Spanish model of colonial government. Spain's interest in her colonies was singularly extractive and geared toward exploiting the natural and human resources of these territories. As such, Spanish government in Latin America involved no model of a social contract, provided little or nothing in the way of services to the native population, and often hampered national economic development by imposing mercantilist trade policies and high taxes on any productive activity. Under colonial rule, government posts were often dispensed as sinecures and petty graft became an unquestioned and universal dimension of colonial life. In 1898 an American observer described municipal Spanish administrators in Cuba as, "pitifully bad; their constant aim being to do as little work as possible and to enrich themselves, at the cost of Cuba, as quickly as they could" (Porter, 1899:11). Cuba's early republican leaders often appeared to repeat this pattern. As one dismayed Cuban patriot stated in 1925,

> Nearly every public evil from which we [Cubans] suffered during the Spanish regime, and against which we so bitterly protested from the platform in the press, and on the battlefield, we have perpetuated *of our own free will* under the Republic. Indeed we have in many cases aggravated these evils (Roig, 1925:513, emphasis added).

There was, however, one key difference between the Cuba (the Republic) and Cuba (the Spanish colony). Whereas Spain's oppressive colonial rule was more or less fixed and stable, the electoral politics of the early Platt era meant that any aspiring *caudillo* could seize power by manipulating elections. Correspondingly, the Platt Amendment meant that any *caudillo* savvy enough to manipulate the United States into intervening in Cuban on his behalf could also take control of the country (and the national treasury). Violence, electoral fraud, and the deliberate manipulation of U.S. imperial intervention all became constant themes in Cuban politics in the Platt era, along with widespread political corruption and graft. Between 1902 and 1933 there were at least eight unsuccessful insurrections (1903, 1907, 1910, 1912, 1924, 1931, 1934, and 1935) in Cuba, three successful "revolutions" (1906, 1917, 1933) and four U.S. political/military interventions (1906, 1917, 1921, and 1933). Furthermore, each of these U.S. interventions was actively solicited by one or more of Cuba's warring political factions.

All of these dynamics had important implications for public health and sanitation efforts. In Cuba's early *caudillo* regimes, political followers were rewarded with jobs through which they were allowed to enrich themselves via embezzlement and petty extortion. In return for these privileges, they were also expected to use their official powers to attack rival political leaders. Concessions for public improvements offered particularly lucrative areas of graft and patronage, and whenever a new *caudillo* managed to seize power in Cuba one of his first actions was inevitably to nullify the public works contracts of his predecessors, and award them instead to his own political allies (who typically pocketed most of the funds). Many public works projects were begun during these years, but few were completed, and health often suffered as a result.

The Graft Clique and the Revolution of 1906

Cuba's first president, Tómas Estrada Palma, was elected prior to the departure of United States troops in 1902. In the eyes of U.S. political and military leaders, the Estrada Palma administration began the political life of the new republic in an ideal situation, and many North Americans expressed high hopes for Cuba's future peace and prosperity under his rule. In a letter to New York in 1902, General Leonard Wood wrote,

> The government of Cuba started off with every preparation made so far as we could foresee which would tend to make a good government possible. The machine is in good running order. In fact the whole matter must now rest with the Cubans themselves. Certainly no nation ever started off under conditions such as Cuba has started with. All departments thoroughly organized; public buildings as a rule renovated and equipped; and a good balance in the Treasury. . . . If there is any failure, it must be charged to the people who follow us (Letter from Leonard Wood to A.B. Farquhar, New York June 1, 1902)

Unfortunately, North American policy makers failed to grasp the economic motivations of Cuba's aspiring politicians, and thus did not anticipate how quickly the "disgruntled political aspirants" who were not part of the Estrada Palma administration would organize a rebellion. A small insurrection took place in Oriente Province less than a year after the withdrawal of U.S. troops. By 1906 this movement had grown into a significant rebellion by the opposition party against the rule of Moderate Party President Tomás Estrada Palma.

These rebellions were provoked in part by the tendency of Cuba's *caudillo*-politicians to seek exclusive personal control over the public sector and the lucrative graft opportunities that came with public office. Some of the dynamics of this patronage system were revealed in a series of affidavits filed by an individual named Woolsey Field in 1907. In these documents, Field details a number of lucrative financial arrangements between officials of the Estrada Palma administration and certain key North American businessmen (termed the "graft clique") who had previously assisted the Cuban independence movement. These businessmen were allegedly rewarded by their Cuban political allies with monopoly concessions in such lucrative industries such as railways, public works contracts, electricity and real estate development.

The Cuban politicians, in turn, were rewarded with substantial kickbacks.

Frank Steinhart was one of the key businessmen named in Field's critical exposé. Steinhart had been a soldier in the U.S. army and served as chief clerk under General Brook during the military occupation of Cuba. The United States Army left him in charge of its archival records from the occupation, and he continued to serve as a liaison between political leaders in Washington, DC and Havana for many years.

Steinhart was able to use these contacts to create a business empire for himself in Cuba, and he eventually held controlling shares in the Havana Electric Company, and served as a broker for multimillion dollar loans arranged between New York banks and the new Cuban government. He held additional interests in Polar Brewery, Allianza insurance, La Cubana insurance and served as President of Jockey Club. Steinhart was the first president of the American Chamber of Commerce in Cuba when it was founded in 1919, and according to one observer in the 1920s, served as "the power behind the scenes who named governments elected presidents and above all was the high intelligence which maintained for years the necessary liaison between the U.S. and Cuba, both political and commercial . . . " Woon (1929:167). In Field's affidavit, Steinhart is described as one of the men "through whom all business with the [Cuban] government must pass."

Norman Davis, T.L. Huston and Horatio Rubens were also named as key members of the graft clique that monopolized business concessions during the Estrada Palma administration. Davis and Huston were partners together with Carlos Manuel de Cespedes in a public works project to dredge the Havana harbor in 1904. Together they developed several affiliated corporations, the Huston Concrete Company and the Huston-Trumbo Dredging Company. They also acquired the Camoa quarry near Havana. One individual noted in 1912, "No other foreign concern outside the great railway corporations has had as great a share in the building up of modern Cuba [as the Huston group]" (quoted in Jenks, 1928:121).

The significance of the patronage system described by Woolsey Field goes beyond mere allegations of corruption in the Estrada Palma administration. The phenomenon Field was describing involves a complex fusion of political power with economic interests that would go on to affect party politics in Cuba throughout the Platt era. More importantly, the clique excluded members of the rival Liberal party from participation in graft, providing a powerful economic motivation for the Liberals to oust Estrada Palma from power. The constraints of the Platt Amendment, however, meant that aspiring office-seekers could not seize power by force outright, but instead had to motivate the United States to intervene on their behalf.

To increase the likelihood of a U.S. intervention, Liberal Party rebels strategically targeted North American sugar plantations for arson prior to the elections of 1906. These aspiring *caudillos* reasoned that attacks on American property would prompt quick retaliation by American armed forces against the Estrada Palma government for its inability to secure property rights, a situation that would favor the Liberals (Wright, 1910). By August 1906, the situation had deteriorated into open rebellion and violence between the two political parties, and President Palma—essentially helpless with his meager guard force—petitioned the United States for help to quell the insurrection. The Liberals simultaneously petitioned the United States to intervene under the Platt Amendment and oust Estrada Palma for his dictatorial seizure of power after excluding them from participation in the national government.

The Second U.S. Intervention, 1906–1909

President Roosevelt was reluctant to intervene in Cuba and ignored the first cables from Estrada Palma requesting U.S. aid in resolving the situation. It was only after a series of extremely urgent cables from Frank Steinhart (who himself may have had questionable motives) stating that the fragile American experiment in state-building was tottering on the verge of anarchy did Roosevelt consent to send Secretary of State Robert Bacon together Secretary of War William Taft to Cuba to investigate the disturbance.

The second U.S. military occupation of Cuba thus occurred at the urging of both political parties in Cuba, who sought United States arbitration in a growing civil conflict that was motivated primarily by a quest for political office and exclusion from graft opportunities. In fact, the bitterness and factionalism between parties was so intense during this time that several noted Cuban politicians stated they would prefer to see Cuba in the hands of the U.S. military than in the hands of the opposing political party—in other words, military occupation by a foreign power was preferable to national independence under the rule of their political enemies (described in Guggenheim, 1934).

Shortly after U.S. troops landed in 1906, the army sent a number of officers out to local provinces to survey popular opinions about local political issues. Frequently the individuals interviewed for these reports welcomed the U.S. troops and lobbied for an extended military occupation as a means to prevent such conflicts from evolving in the future. One military report from Oriente Province described an interview with a local planter who stated, "[T]he longer Americans stay the better it will be for Cuba . . . after the Liberals win many of them will join moderates, because there will not be enough offices to go around." Another report from Oriente described local sentiment in favor of U.S. occupation or annexation,

> The three brothers [all members of a wealthy family of sugar planters] agree in their views on the political situation. They ardently desire annexation, but admit that they, like other Cubans of property, are afraid to express their opinions openly because their property will be destroyed should the U.S. leave here. They say a protectorate, or at least U.S. supervision of affairs is necessary to prevent anarchy (Confidential report to Charles Magoon from Capt. Crain, Oriente Province, Feb 2, 1907).

Since Cuba had no functioning national government at the time of the 1906 elections, the United States established a provisional administration under the control of Charles Magoon (former governor of the Canal Zone in Panama) from 1906 until 1909. Magoon immediately put the U.S. army to work once again building roads, correcting lapses in sanitation and constructing ambitious public works project. According to Jenks (1928:99) "Magoon built in two years almost as many kilometers of roads as had been built in the four centuries preceding."

In Oriente province, the occupying army also instituted new sanitation measures that greatly curbed the incidence of malaria. According to Lindsey (1911:205), " A determined and systematic campaign has been waged against the anopheles, or malaria mosquitoes. As a result, malaria, which Cubans look upon as a necessary evil, has been reduced to a negligible quantify." In 1903 a local mining company in Oriente reported that on average at least 83 percent of its workforce was sick with malaria at some point during the year. After the imposition of mosquito control measures by the U.S. army during Magoon's term as provisional governor, the rate dropped to 17 percent (in 1909) (reported in Lindsey, 1911:205).

One of Magoon's most pressing tasks during this time were to sort out the nature of the conflict between the rival political parties, and to reinforce Cuba's legal codes and constitution to insure that a similar breakdown of authority would not happen in the future. To try and arbitrate between Cuba's warring political factions, Magoon established a committee of leading Liberals representing those excluded by Estrada Palma, and allowed them to petition him as provisional governor. A problem developed almost immediately when the Liberal party itself fell apart into two warring factions—those united around Santa Clara strongman Jose Miguel Gómez, and those in favor of the less charismatic Alfredo Zayas. In a confidential letter to William Howard Taft, Magoon stated,

> . . . The campaigns of both Zayas and Gómez have been, and are being conducted on the basis of the ability of each chieftain to provide his adherents with offices or some form of governmental employment . . . The feeling between the two factions is very bitter. Each tries to have every vacancy filled by one of his partisans and failing in that exerts himself equally to prevent the vacancy being filled . . . each side promises anything and everything for the support of individuals or groups, and it would be quite impossible for either one to "make good" on even a small percentage of his promises (Magoon to Taft, July 21, 1907).

This split in the Liberal Party well illustrates the inherent instability of Cuba's political coalitions. These groups were not formed out of ideological differences, but by vertical hierarchies of patron-client relations coalescing and fragmenting around a common desire to share in the spoils of war. Even Woolsey Field, whose damning affidavits describing the "graft clique" of the Estrada Palma regime, was not actually an impartial observer, but an active agent in political intrigue acting on behalf of the Zayas faction. According to several reports, Field was paid to publicize his knowledge of the Moderate Party graft clique by a coalition that included Alfredo Zayas along with several North American capitalists who were seeking to discredit President Roosevelt. The key lesson to draw from Woolsey Field's affidavits, therefore, is not that there was graft and corruption in the new Cuban republic, but that certain ambitious individuals were excluded from these lucrative arrangements and used that exclusion as a reason to foment the "revolution" (and subsequent U.S. intervention) of 1906.

North American planters also sought to manipulate the United States into intervening in Cuba under the provisions of the Platt Amendment to protect themselves from the extortion demands of Cuba's avaricious *caudillos*. In October, 1907 a *New York Times* reporter interviewed a North American sugar planter in Cuba who spoke openly of intentionally creating "disturbances" or even "revolutions" to manipulate the United States into intervening in Cuba,

> For $500, said the [American] planter with a grin, I can raise a disturbance of some kind which will cause talk in the United States. For $5,000 I can organize a revolution, and you fellows might as well understand now as any other time that whenever you propose to leave us to the tender mercies of these Spanish-American bandits a mysterious revolution will break out somewhere in the island which will necessitate your immediate intervention [under the Platt Amendment] (quoted in the *New York Times*, October 23, 1907).

It is important to note that the "Spanish-American bandits" the planter is referring to were not bandits in the traditional sense, but the various Cuban political coalitions who sought to extort money from planters. These extortion attempts occurred on multiple levels. Existing office holders imposed high taxes for purposes of graft and corruption, and out-of-power insurgents sought to fund antigovernment insurrections by extorting funds from wealthy planters (most often by threatening to burn cane fields). All public employees, even schoolteachers were forced to contribute money to political leaders. According to one report, "Señor Panades the head of the Educational Board in this city [Camaguey], has compelled all the teachers to be assessed and pay 10 percent of their month's salary for the Campaign Funds for the Liberal party" (Memo to Magoon from John Furlong, November 11, 1908). North American planters were a minority at this time, and as such were frequently targeted for a practice described by one scholar as "bureaucratic extortion of pariah capital"(Scott, 1972). In other words, North American citizens attempting to do business in Cuba without strong political protection were subject to arbitrary taxation and fines by Cuba's personalistic judiciary.

A number of North American planters homesteading on the Isle of Pines wrote letters to U.S. officials protesting these petty extortion activities on the part of Cuban officials. In 1906 a group of Americans sent the following complaint to Charles Magoon at the beginning of the second U.S. military occupation of Cuba,

> The correctional judge [on the Isle of Pines] has never failed to have an American arrested on the slightest possible charge and in almost every instance has given him the extreme limit of penalty prescribed by the law and in some cases has supplied both the law and penalty himself. One American was arrested and fined $45.00 for repairing a public road in front of his place, which had become impassable. The authorities had refused to make the repair and as the debris was forcing the water over his farm he undertook to repair the same at his own expense but after spending much time and money thereon was arrested and fined $45.00. . . . In conclusion we would respectfully say that for more than four years past that the American residents of this Island have stood with commendable patience the injustice and arrogance of these officials, who are still performing the functions of their respective offices and in the same manner as formerly and we desire to especially emphasize the fact, that it is these same officials, who are more directly responsible for the strained condition existing on the island in the past and at the present moment than any other cause (letter from Charles Raynard, Secretary, American Federation of the Isle of Pines, to Hon. Edwin V. Morgan, Minister Plenipoteniary, Havana, Cuba October 24, 1906).

Caudillo Politics and Health Decline, 1902–1906

Upon taking control of Cuba in 1906 Provisional Governor Charles Magoon described health conditions in Havana as generally positive, but noted that sanitation efforts in the interior of the island were "practically nil." Magoon went on to attribute the deterioration on health in interior towns to neglect on the part of local political leaders. In an early report to Washington, DC Magoon stated, "These towns, aided by the State, spent millions annually in sanitation, but it was ineffective because the sanitary officials were subject to local [political] influences, and did not enforce the laws"(Magoon, report to W.H. Taft, August 10, 1907).

Detailed statistical records from this era are not available[2], but many reports from this time period confirm Magoon's observations of declines in health and sanitation outside of Havana following the withdrawal of U.S. troops from Cuba in 1902. At this time, and in keeping with the Spanish colonial model, elected officials (including health officials) in the provinces tended to view government positions as sinecures to be distributed on the basis of political loyalty. This patronage system led to a general inertia in the public sector with respect to health and sanitation measures, and a tendency for local officials to pocket funds allocated for health improvements. Members of local health departments were also encouraged by their superiors to issue citations only to members of the opposing political party. The violence and instability caused by power struggles between rival *caudillos* also drained economic resources from the state government and left health programs greatly underfunded.

In 1907 and 1909 the *New York Times* ran articles describing sanitary neglect in Cuba. In 1907 the newspaper charged that a significant resurgence of yellow fever in Cienfuegos resulted from neglect and mismanagement of the water supply (*New York Times*, September 30, 1907). In 1909 these allegations were repeated with much stronger wording,

> There were no cases of yellow fever for some time after the United States turned the control of the island's affairs over to President Palma. But the Cubans cared little for the work that had been done by the Americans, and at the time of the second intervention in the fall of 1906 there had been several cases of yellow fever on the island. It took the American experts a long time to root out the disease for the second time. Now it appears that the Cubans are following their old policy of neglect again, with the practical certainty that before long there will be a recurrence of yellow fever in Havana, with all its consequent danger to the neighboring cities in the United States (*New York Times*, May 29, 1909).

The dynamics of health decline in Oriente province following the withdrawal of U.S. troops in 1902 were described in a series of private letters sent from Antonio Zamorro, the provincial sanitation officer in Oriente Province under the U.S. military occupation, to both the provincial governor and the Cuban President between 1903–1905. In these letters Zamorro frequently complains of deficiencies in both resources and political will to enforce sanitation decrees put in place during the Occupation. He noted that during the U.S. occupation the average amount spent by the American army on sanitation per month in the city of Santiago was approximately $8,849. In the first year of Republican government under President Tomás Estrada Palma this figure was reduced to $4,788, and by 1905 it had fallen as low as $1,200 per month—an 85 percent reduction in spending (Antonio Zamorro to Provincial governor of Oriente Province and President Tómas Estrada Palma, 1903; 1905). This shortage of funds was also greatly compounded by the problem of allocation, and Zamorro also implied in his letters that funds designated for public health were often pocketed by corrupt administrators.

Even more importantly, it appears that in Oriente province there was a critical breakdown in public health enforcement authority. Without the occupying army or a stable federal government to coerce compliance, many people (municipal authorities included) simply ignored the citations of the sanitary commissioner. In one series of appeals from Zamorro to the provincial governor, for instance, he complained that the mayor of El Cristo (a small town outside of Santiago) continually refused to dispose of a horse that had died next to the town's train station, despite numerous citations. "I begged first, and finally ordered the mayor of the town [to dispose of the decaying horse] . . . After innumerable excuses and pretexts he went and, in a scarcely discernible manner, put a little gasoline and some dry grass on top [of the horse to try and incinerate it], leaving it in worse condition than before, as it had begun to rain."

What this example reveals is comparative inefficiency of civilian verses military government in matters of sanitation, and the tradeoffs in terms of health and sanitation that inevitably occur following a transition to a factionalized, personalistic government. During the U.S. occupation, for instance, animal disposal would have been organized by the military, and executed in a timely and disciplined manner. The penalties for noncompliance were severe. In a highly personalistic civilian government, however, (especially one that was only one year old and had not yet had time to consolidate its authority), such unpleasant tasks could effectively be avoided through passive resistance. While this might represent a subjective improvement from the civilian population's point of view (i.e., they were no longer subject to unwanted foreign occupation or repressive military measures), it was not beneficial for public health.

Sanitary commissioner Zamorro naturally felt quite frustrated by the political inertia he perceived in the municipal government, and began a series of impassioned appeals to the provincial governor and to President Estrada Palma warning of serious health consequences if the situation were allowed to deteriorate further. In September, 1903 Zamorro wrote to President Palma:

> Sanitation merits special consideration, but disgracefully, it has in this city, fallen into a deficient state in both the personnel and material needed to complete its humanitarian and patriotic mission. For the resources the local government has provided are very scarce, and . . . certain important elements [meaning municipal government] have made it impossible, day by day, to keep the city clean.

This letter initiated a series of increasingly bitter confrontations between Antonio Zamorro and local Santiago officials who resented the way Zamorro continually implicated them in charges of mismanagement. When Zamorro was discovered to be circulating leaflets criticizing his superiors for their general inattention to public health, he was promptly fired for "failure to comply with orders, irregular conduct, and insubordination" (Mayor of Santiago to Provincial Governor of Oriente Province, 1904). Zamorro was briefly reinstated, then later replaced with a less zealous, and more politically aware sanitary commissioner.

Members of the Liberal Party also protested to Charles Magoon that the Department of Public Works in Havana was used as a political instrument by the Conservative-Moderate Party under Estrada Palma. Street cleaners were expected to follow the dictates of the Party, and even to serve on occasion as an armed brigade to keep Liberal voters from participating in national elections. In one report to Magoon it was noted that,

> Hundreds of workmen are employed, perhaps thousands, [in Havana] in sweeping the streets and washing them and caring for the gardens and parks and transporting garbage. . . . It is necessary to be a Moderate [party member] in order to be a street sweeper, that has been organized in this City in a most marvelous way, so that on the 23 of Sept, 1905 the elections in Havana were won by Moderate street sweepers in this way. About 11 am a troop of laborers, or of street sweepers were employed and together with all employees from the Department of Public Works and all parts of the service were taken to the Arsenal where there was a deposits of arms of the Government at that time. They were all armed and distributed through the City through which they galloped firing their arms and ordering the doors of houses to be closed and threatening away the electors from the precincts. This happened in Santiago and in other places. . . . This

was done with the aggravating circumstances that they were assisted by the Rural Guards in order to impede the Liberals from voting and on the other hand the same men voted in different precincts (Magoon, Charles (undated) Report of Conference between the Provisional Governor and a Commission of the Revolutionary or Liberal Party).

Similar dynamics were described for other public works departments across the island. Jobs with road construction crews and other major infrastructure improvements were used to secure party followers with patronage and graft, and to engage in partisan attacks on political rivals. One report from the town of Trinidad detailed how the city's chief Liberal leader (Panades) corrupted the public health department and destroyed the city's water supply with his political maneuvering,

> The trouble commenced in the city water works, a small pumping station which supplies the city with water, by Panades insisting upon giving positions to certain of his followers who knew nothing about the work and as a result the engine broke down, the engineer resigned as they refused to appoint competent persons to assist him and as a result the city has been without a permanent water supply since then . . . As a result of this condition the city is without water and there is no fuel to run the engines at the pumping station, all the cisterns are practically dry owing to the long drought and the city is threatened with a very unsanitary condition. . . . This city has been considered the healthiest place in the island, there having been no disease here of any kind since the intervention of 1898, but unless they are given a competent government here the former conditions cannot exist, no sanitary laws have been carried out as recommended as there is no one to enforce them and the city is without water. I have telegraphed for authority to purchase the necessary fuel to supply the engines and our men will run the pumps and supply the city and ourselves until a satisfactory government with force enough to carry out necessary measures is established. There is practically no one in recognized authority here with whom I can deal, and were it not for our presence I do not believe there would be any order. Panades, as I have stated, is crazy, and irresponsible, and hopes to put himself in authority and become mayor, this I think would be inadvisable (Letter to Charles Magoon from Company K, 1st Provisional Regiment, U.S.M.C., Trinidad, Cuba March 19, 1907)

One of the most thoroughly documented case of corruption of public health and public works initiatives involved contracts for the construction of a new waterworks and sewage system for the city of Cienfuegos in the early 1900s. The water system in this city had been painfully inadequate since the mid-1800s, but the Spanish had little interest in public works improvements during the colonial period, especially during the violent wars of independence that characterized the latter part of the nineteenth century. By the time of the second U.S. military intervention, Cienfuegos was described as "a standing menace" to international commerce (Clarence Edwards, confidential cable to Charles Magoon, May, 1908). Epidemics of water borne diseases were common in the city, and at least twelve people died in the winter of 1906 from a typhoid outbreak (Charles Magoon, memo to Taft, June 1908).

Constructing a new water and sewer system for the city of Cienfuegos, however, was rendered virtually impossible by the intensity of local political rivalries. Each *caudillo* was determined to defeat any public works or public health project that might benefit his rivals or allow them to gain political leverage via graft and patronage. Just as other Cuban leaders swore they would rather see Cuba under U.S. occupation rather than in the hands of political rivals, it appeared the local politicians in Cienfuegos preferred to have the city endure epidemics of typhoid and waterborne diseases rather than see their rivals benefit from the patronage and graft that would accompany the construction of a new aqueduct. According to one report sent from William Howard Taft to President Roosevelt in 1908,

... The city of Cienfuegos has for forty years been attempting to secure a water and sewer system, but these attempts have always failed because of the high partisan spirit existing between the two political factions in the city, each of which seemed to prefer to defeat the enterprise rather than to permit the other to have charge or supervision of its execution. ..The history of Cienfuegos shows that the partisan spirit which has been rife there for forty years past has prevented and will continue to prevent the construction of the waterworks and sewers by the city government which is always under the control of one or the other of the two warring factions.

In March of 1906, just prior to the second U.S. intervention in Cuba, the municipal government of Cienfuegos arranged for Hugh J. Reilly, a North American contractor, to construct a new waterworks for the city. At the time, the city council was dominated by Conservative/Moderate Party leaders who employed considerable violence to insure the passage of this lucrative project. At least one individual was murdered during the deliberations, and according to one observer, "Frias [the Moderate Party *caudillo*] took advantage of that murder and the excitement it caused to keep the town in a state of terror to hold the referendum vote relating to the loan [for the waterworks] . . . " (Statement from Mr. Leopoldo Figueroa, of Cienfuegos to Charles Magoon March 25, 1908).

When the second U.S. military occupation of Cuba began a few months later, the Conservative-Moderate Cienfuegos city council was dissolved by Charles Magoon and replaced with a new council that included a number of Liberal Party politicians. One of the first actions of this new council was to retract the Reilly contracts on the basis of "illegality." The newly empowered Liberals charged (correctly) that "violence and fraud" had been employed by the Conservative Party leaders to secure the contract with Reilly (Confidential Report to Charles Magoon, May 1908). The Liberals instead sought to award the contract to one of their loyal supporters. This plan was thwarted, however, when Reilly successfully petitioned Charles Magoon and the State Department with documents showing that his original contract had been approved by the provincial governor. After much prolonged negotiation between Washington, DC Havana and the municipality of Cienfuegos, a compromise was finally reached whereby the work would be completed by Reilly, but funded primarily from the national, rather than the municipal treasury.[3] A confidential memorandum sent to Magoon from one of his officers in Cienfuegos detailed the attitudes of local residents regarding these developments,

> . . . [I]n answer to general question what they [the residents of Cienfuegos] thought the best method [of completing the waterworks] almost without exception [they] declared the central government will do work quicker and better through public works, thus depriving [local] political rings opportunity for graft and attendant political power. Reilly rights and interests are not understood wholly nor concerned with but . . . a general acknowledgment of his possessing rights and it was suggested in most cases that government should compromise and settle them. . . . The Conservative party who are followers of Frias strongly advocates the carrying out of Reilly contract as modified, Zayaistas [one faction of the Liberal Party] strongly supported the action of the municipality [in dissolving the contracts and rewarding them to a Liberal party supporter]. Miguelistas [the other faction of the Liberal Party] expressed the opinion that the people desire

water however it may be brought. These are expressions of political ring-leaders only. There is general ignorance amongst the rank and file on status and history of Reilly concession and complete lack of interest . . .

In response to these (and other) complaints about the intense politicization of municipal public works and public health programs during the Estrada Palma administration, Charles Magoon passed a decree placing all public health and sanitation programs under the control of a national health department. This decree abolished local boards and established a National Board of Sanitation that appointed officers for each municipality. The municipalities were required to pay one tenth of their revenues to the national government to defray the cost of the sanitation services (Lockmiller, 1938). Magoon's plan for centralization of health services, however, ultimately proved unsuccessful. As a result, the time period from the end of the second U.S. military occupation in 1909 until the abrogation of the Platt Amendment in 1933 was characterized by deepening cycles of *caudillo* violence and corruption in Cuban politics, with public health and welfare often suffering as a result.

Notes

1. It is impossible to cite all of the works that detail these dynamics. An abbreviated list would include the personal correspondence of U.S. political and military leaders such as Elihu Root, William Howard Taft, Charles Magoon, and Leonard Wood. Journalistic accounts include: Wright (1910), Lindsey (1911), Bonsal (1912), Spinden (1920) and Beals (1934). Leading Cuban nationalists and intellectuals such as Francisco Figureas (1906), Emilio Roig de Leuschenring (1925) and Fernando Ortiz (1927) also echoed these themes in their early writings. Even the early pro-Castro writings of Herbert Matthews in the *New York Times* described office-seeking as the root cause of political violence in Cuba prior to 1959.
2. The provisional government of Cuba under Charles Magoon did collect some health statistics but some key information is missing from these archival records. The health reports of the Magoon's provisional government only cover the time period between October 1907 and July 1908. There are reports on infectious diseases, but they do not specify whether the numbers cited are for individual cases of a certain disease or represent the number of deaths from that disease for a given month. These reports give the general impression that yellow fever had returned Cuba (a total of about twenty cases or deaths were recorded between October and July), and that waterborne diseases remained a serious threat to health. Over one hundred cases (or deaths) of typhoid were reported between October and July. Tuberculosis, measles and diphtheria also continued to pose

threats. These reports also illustrate that despite ongoing problems with infectious disease, Cuba remained a much healthier place than it had been during the War years.

3. This plan also proved unsuccessful. Several years later, President Gómez passed a law barring foreign contractors from bidding on Cuban public works projects, a move that insured that graft dollars would remain in local hands, to be distributed as patronage (reported in the *New York Times*, September 3, 1912).

8

Caudillismo, Instability and Health Trends in the Platt Era, 1909–1933

It is difficult to accurately assess health trends in Cuba during the remainder of the Platt era. The escalating intensity of Cuba's *caudillo* wars meant that each political faction used increasingly aggressive tactics to try and persuade the United States to intervene under the Platt Amendment and remove the existing leader from power. Given that Article Five of the Platt Amendment allowed for intervention if Cuba failed to maintain appropriate health and sanitation programs, rival *caudillos* frequently accused one another of allowing sanitation to lapse and thus risking another military occupation by the United States.

To defend themselves from these attacks, *caudillos* in office took great care to produce favorable national health statistics, ostensibly reflecting great progress and humanitarian achievement during their rule. The ritual recitation of these sanitation accomplishments to visiting journalists and American public health professionals served a dual purpose of discrediting the previous regime (i.e., the rivals who had fled to Miami and were trying to organize another intervention or coup), and diverting attention away from the dictatorial exercise of power and personalism that typically characterized their rule. Exiled "revolutionary juntas," on the other hand, countered by accusing the regime in power of endangering the health and sovereignty of the Republic by provoking another U.S. intervention under article five of the Platt Amendment.

In other words, it is possible to find completely contradictory health statistics and claims for nearly every Cuban president from 1909 to the present. Government publications from each administration report on great advances in health care, the establishment of new hospitals and progress in the control of infectious and parasitic diseases (LeRoy y Cassá, 1913; Lopez de Valle, 1924; Guiteras, 1962; Lopez Silvero, 1926; 1930; Fernandez, 1930; Silvero, 1930; Secretaria de Sanidad y Beneficencia, 1931; Ministerio de Salubridad y Asistencia Social, 1953; MINISAP, 1960; MINISAP, 1969; MINISAP, 1979; Dominguez, 1987). Revolutionary juntas and out-of-power coalitions, on the other hand, describe neglected sanitation programs, resurgent epidemics, graft and corruption in the management of health resources by the government (Cuban Information Bureau, 1931; Beals, 1934; Batista, 1964; Batista, 1962; Castellanos, 1962a; Castellanos, 1962b; The Cuban Report, 1964; Castellanos, 1963).

Under these circumstance, both government publications and exile propaganda must be viewed with some degree of skepticism. Unfortunately, all of the original archival records from Cuba's Health Ministry from this time period were destroyed in 1933 when radical students bombed the government office that contained the documents (*New York Times*, February 7, 1933). Several alternative sources of information are available from these years, but they often lack the temporal continuity necessary to accurately document changes in health over time. One United States Public Health Service office remained open in Havana after 1911, but these reports are often incomplete.[1]

The Cuban Academy of Sciences occasionally published internal papers on health and sanitation during this period. Given that these papers were intended for a very small internal audience of (nonpolitical) Cuban academics they may be taken as reasonably scientific and unpoliticized. *The New York Times* (and other major North American newspapers) maintained bureaus in Cuba and often reported on newsworthy health events (such as epidemic disease) that might affect North American travelers or tourists to the island. There were also several independent American writers and journalists living in Cuba at this time, who were not affiliated with either the Cuban or American government who published independent accounts of Cuban politics and health. And finally, there are a few archival sources that contain private correspondence between provincial sanitation offices and government officials.

These alternative sources, if taken individually, do not necessarily constitute a formidable challenge to official declarations of the various

Cuban Ministries of Health and Sanitation, but when viewed collectively, as mutually corroborating testimony, contradict many government reports and offer credibility to charges of a consistent pattern of public health neglect and decline during the Platt era. In other words, these alternative sources suggest that most Cuban leaders viewed public health and public works departments in terms of opportunities for graft and patronage, and that health often suffered as a result. Because of the threat of U.S. intervention under Article Five of the Platt Amendment, however, it appears each ruler deliberately released favorable health propaganda to divert attention from these lapses.

The Gómez Regime, 1909–1912

The second United States military occupation of Cuba was brought to a close with the inauguration of José Miguel Gómez (of the Liberal Party) in January, 1909. For the purposes of the election, the Gómez and Zayas factions of the Liberals had reunited in an uneasy truce with Zayas as vice-president. William Howard Taft was also elected President of the United States in 1909, and having witnessed first hand the problems brought by the "revolution" of 1906, expressed no further desire to intervene in Cuba under the Platt Amendment during his tenure as president.

Gómez, aware of Taft's unwillingness to intervene, soon revealed himself to be a typical *caudillo*. According to Chapman (1927:302) "Once in office . . . he [Gómez] showed the normal . . . tendency to dominate all branches of the government." This domination extended to the national treasury and to the military, both of which were placed under Gómez' personal control. While the exact amount embezzled by Gómez during his term of office is unknown, it was frequently observed at the time that he entered politics as a bankrupt farmer, and left a multimillionaire. Upon leaving office he built a $250,000 marble palace on the Prado in Havana, and was estimated to have at least $8 million invested in mines and sugar. His salary as president was $25,000 a year (*The Independent*, July 19, 1924).

Gómez did not just appropriate treasury funds for his personal use. He also inflated all areas of government spending by handing out sinecures[2] to his followers to insure their loyalty. To fund these extravagant expenditures, a $16 million loan was contracted with Speyer and Company, a North American banking group. The ostensible purpose of the loan was for public works improvements across the island, but most of the money was diverted to building up a new army and handing out *botellas*.

Under Gómez' rule, the post of secretary of sanitation in the Cuban cabinet became increasingly used as a political appointment to harass members of the opposing party for sanitary infractions. This practice prompted outcries from many noted Cuban scientists. Dr. Juan Guiteras, a Cuban physician second in fame only to Carlos Finlay, resigned his post as director of sanitation under President Gómez to protest the increasing politicization of public health (Exposito, 1947). According to one Cuban historian (Exposito, 1947), "As a general rule, these men [political appointments in public health] represented elements who didn't want to work, but to enjoy the wealth of the state. The eternal curse of politics had become the cancer of public health administration."

The military buildup under Gómez also constituted a serious drain on government finances. In 1905 President Estrada Palma had governed Cuba with only a rural guard force of 3000 men. Under Magoon's administration, the rural guard had been increased to a total of 5,180 men—a number judged by U.S. officials to be sufficient to maintain order. Gómez, however, created an entire new infantry brigade in addition to the rural guard which raised the total number of soldiers in Cuba to 10,000 by 1910, and to over 15,000 by 1912 (Chapman, 1927:390).

Given that Cuba had no enemies and was not at war in the early 1900s, this military buildup was described by several observers as an attempt by Gómez to consolidate his power by creating a personal military force. These troops were not intended to promote public order or attack enemy nations but to extort money from Cuban citizens via petty graft, and to harass and attack members of the opposition party. The rural guard, for instance, had been created to serve under President Estrada Palma, a member of the Conservative Party. Gómez, a Liberal, did not trust them to protect his interests and instead sought to build up a separate armed force of Liberal supporters, in part to attack the Conservatives and the rural guard. The existence of rival partisan armies in Cuba would go on to create decades of violence and low intensity civil conflict. As Lindsey (1911:148) described,

The keenest rivalry and the bitterest feeling exist between the rural guard [built up by Estrada Palma and the Conservative party] and the regular army [build up by Gómez and the his branch of the Liberal Party]. In a case of civil war, these bodies would surely take opposite sides, and neither has any loyalty to the flag, or allegiance to the government. The chief influence to which they would be amenable is the will of their respective commanders, who are politicians and aim to employ the forces under them as political instruments.

Caudillismo and Militarization

These dynamics illustrate a key feature of *caudillo* rule. In these regimes the security forces of the state are not a neutral or impartial body but are viewed as a personal security force used to establish and police the *caudillo*'s claim on the country's economic resources. Whenever a new leader took control of Cuba (either by force or via elections), one of his first actions was always to replace the existing leaders of the police and army and install his own loyal followers instead. Rivals were imprisoned or driven into exile.

In the early years of the republic, Cuba's *caudillos* also established a pattern of using amnesty bills to exempt their own followers from criminal penalties. A total of sixteen such laws were passed in the Cuban senate between 1902 and 1923. According to Chapman (1927:524),

> The majority of those who received the favor of these laws were the worst sort of criminals, who for political reasons (to assist congressmen in retaining their posts) were allowed to escape the penalties they had incurred. . . . The protection afforded by Congress to members of its own body committing crimes, through the interpretation given to congressional immunity [meant that] . . . as a result, there was no law which congressmen and their friends need obey.

The key lesson to draw from these amnesty and immunity bills is not so much one of moral outrage that crime was excused for politicians and their followers, *but that these criminal acts remained prohibited for the rest of the population.* As a result, elected officials were able to obtain a virtual monopoly in Havana's lucrative vice trades since these activities remained prohibited for ordinary citizens. Cuba's politicians effectively used criminal penalties to establish and protect their economic territory. Out of power *caudillos*, on the other hand, would often assert themselves by challenging the established economic territory of those in power. This would inevitably lead to arrest and imprisonment, since those in power used criminal penalties to protect their market control. Almost every Cuban president between 1902 and 1959, for example, was either imprisoned or forced into exile at some point in his political career.[3]

The inevitable consequences of this type of political/economic organization are increased militarization, violence and instability. Between 1910 and 1920 the size of the Cuban army tripled from 10,000 (under Gómez) to over 30,000 (under Machado). According to one observer, "If the United States army were in the same proportion to the population [as the Cuban] it would be six times its present size . . . The inflated army is a political army" (Norton, 1926:81). The size of this (already inflated) army was doubled again in the years after Machado's overthrow, and reached a high of around 45–50,000 in the late 1950s. Given that Cuba had no real enemies at this time, the purpose of this vast military apparatus was primarily to secure and enforce the president's economic monopolies. This practice generated an inevitable tendency for military expansion—a new ruler who seized power had to purge his predecessor's followers from the army and build himself a new, larger army capable of effectively combating the recently demobilized forces of the previous *caudillo*.

With an expanded army, more and more markets could become targeted for takeover. By the 1920s, Cuba had the largest military in proportion to its population in the hemisphere (Norton, 1926). Machado even put meat and milk distribution under monopoly control of the army during his rule (Beals, 1934). This increasing militarization meant that the scope of Cuba's "revolutions" became hugely amplified over time with major segments of the economy and society reconfigured after a new leader seized power.

Rebellion and Resistance under Gómez

Several revolts broke out in Cuba during Gómez' presidency, organized by Conservatives who were angered at losing their opportunities for political graft as well as having become imprisoned and harassed by Liberal Party public officials. These movements involved impassioned petitions to the United States to intervene under the Platt Amendment and oust Gómez from power for his dictatorial excesses, primarily so that the Conservatives could themselves take control of these lucrative political offices. In 1910 a small Conservative revolt was organized near El Canay in Oriente Province, and in 1911, another revolt was led by a disaffected army General in Havana.

The tension between Gómez and Zayas intensified as the 1912 election drew closer. Eventually, Gómez's personal animosity toward his vice-president proved to be much stronger than his loyalty to the Liberal Party—and in retaliation for Zayas' coup attempt, Gómez began secretly began using his control over the military to back the Conservative Party candidate (General Mario Menocal) for office against Zayas.

The key region in deciding the elections turned out to be Oriente Province, and to secure General Menocal's victory, Gómez had his army employ terrorism, blackmail, vote-buying and other forms of electoral fraud throughout Oriente (Chapman, 1927). Electoral violence increased throughout the fall. In October, 1912 (shortly before the national elections) a gunfight erupted between Liberals and Conservatives in Havana's central park, and political meetings across the city resulted in major riots (*New York Times*, October 26, 1912). The police themselves were often Zayas partisans, and their attempts to restore order involved selective prosecution of Conservative activists. The Liberals protested these tactics both at home and abroad (establishing another exile junta in New York), hoping to prompt another American intervention that would settle the "voting irregularities" in their favor, as happened in 1906. Their pleas for intervention were ineffective, however, and in January 1913 Mario Menocal became the third president of the Cuban Republic.

The Menocal Administration (1913–1921)

The same dynamics (graft, patronage, *caudillo* violence) that shaped the Gómez administration again played themselves out in the Menocal presidency—only more intensely. As one report noted, "During the eight years of the Menocal administration . . . the government collected revenues amounting to $600 million; nevertheless General Menocal bequeathed to the country a floating debt of $46 million without having made any substantial contributions to social development" (Commission on Cuban Affairs, 1935:8).

One of Menocal's first acts as President was to install friends and family members into high paying government jobs with no actual service required. He continued the buildup and politicization of the military, and specifically targeted the remaining Liberals for various forms of harassment by the rural guard and police. Reports from the provincial archives in Santiago-de-Cuba reveal that from the time of Menocal's inauguration, many state agencies became employed in partisan ways. Police were sent to monitor and harass Liberal meetings, the sanitation inspector was reported to be issuing citations only to Liberal establishments, and the Rural Guard were permitted to raid plantations of known liberal supporters.

Menocal's abuses of power prompted the leading Liberal in the Senate, Orestes Ferrara to proclaim, "If this state of affairs continues the Liberals will be compelled to withdraw from public life, and as there will be no guarantee for the safety of their lives they will be compelled to resort to revolution" (*New York Times*, April, 15, 1913). Similar occurrences took place in Santa Clara, where the (Conservative Party affiliated) rural guard was accused of using assassination and violence to further the political goals of its leaders. By 1915 it was clear that Menocal intended to use the powers of the presidency (and the coercive force of the Rural Guard) to have himself reelected. The Liberals also remained divided, but Zayas (despite the continued opposition of Gómez) again finagled the nomination for himself. Following Zayas' nomination, Gómez brokered a deal where he would again switch party affiliation again and throw his support to Zayas in exchange for control of various cabinet positions.

Sugar prices peaked at this time, due to the destruction of European beet-fields in World War I. This led the insurgents to burn cane-fields in order to compel American planters to petition the United States for intervention on behalf of the Liberals. Menocal also used the insurrection to expand his powers as executive and he remained a virtual dictator until the end of his term. One of his more effective tactics was to grant incarcerated criminals pardons and turn them loose upon the public on the condition that they would serve as his own personal militia. During his eight years in office, Menocal granted 2,900 pardons, as compared with 1,500 for Gómez (in four years), and 324 for Estrada Palma (in four years) (Perez, 1986:218),

> . . . [M]any criminals were pardoned in 1920 by President Menocal . . . on the understanding that they should earn their freedom by acting as gunmen and bullies for the party of the government. So that the government had at its disposal the corrupt elements of the army, both as military supervisors

and as soldiers, and likewise it had special agents, some of who were pardoned criminals (Spinden, 1920:476).

By his second term of office, Menocal had managed to secure near dictatorial powers for himself, and the Liberal Party had become increasingly disenfranchised. Unable to formally participate in national politics, they responded by fomenting another revolution. By 1917 this conflict had escalated until the country was practically torn in two by the warring factions. At one point, nearly all of Oriente Province was in the hands of the Liberals and over 2,000 Liberal sympathizers took up arms in Santiago against Mencoal's supporters. With the possibility of civil war growing day by day, the United States reluctantly decided to act. U.S. warships carrying sixteen hundred American soldiers were dispatched to Oriente, with the mission of protecting American properties from the violent bands of raiders terrorizing the countryside.

The 1917 insurrection was much more destructive than the previous rebellion in 1912. "Bridges were destroyed, miles of railroad track torn up, telegraph and telephone wires were torn down, putting half of Cuba out of communication with the capital for weeks" (Jenks, 1929:188). American planters in Oriente continued to petition the U.S. government to provide them (and the Cuban sugar crop) with protection. The U.S. wanted to remain impartial, however, and took the position that these problems were internal to Cuba and any intervention in favor of the insurgents would be acting against the "constitutional government." Thus protected by the desire of the imperial power to remain neutral, Menocal was able to consolidate his dictatorial powers and serve a second term.

Given the intractability of the Liberals in Congress, Menocal governed almost exclusively by executive decree during his second term. There was also a huge increase in American investment in Cuba during his administration. Sugar production and economic prosperity increased dramatically, driven by a surge in prices following World War I. By 1919 almost 500,000 acres of Oriente were planted in cane, surpassing the entire Cuban area under cane cultivation in 1899 (Hoernel, 1976). These high sugar prices brought a certain general prosperity to Cuba, but also many potential problems, since much of the development was based on investment of foreign capital.

At the height of the postwar sugar prosperity (known as the "dance of the millions"), over one quarter of Cuba's sugar mills changed hands, with Cuban-owned mills increasingly bought up (at extraordinarily high prices) by large American corporations seeking to consolidate their holdings. Following the Dance of the Millions, sugar prices plummeted sharply, and many of the remaining Cuban owners, who had borrowed heavily from American banks during the boom were suddenly faced with bankruptcy and foreclosure. Unable to pay back their loans, these planters had their lands and mills taken over by American banks. In 1921, the National City Bank of New York alone took over between fifty and sixty Cuban-owned sugar mills, and American corporations ultimately gained control of almost fifty percent of Cuba's mills during this time (Jenks, 1929).

These powerful capitalists (including such financial institutions as J.P. Morgan, the Chase National Bank, National City Bank of New York, and J.W. Seligman) put increasing pressure on the United States to protect them and their Cuban investments by actively employing the Platt Amendment to control Cuban political decision-making. As a result, the U.S. State Department began a program of "prophylactic intervention," reasoning that increasing pressure on Cuban politicians to govern "responsibly" would prevent future insurrections, satisfy American capitalists, and hopefully eliminate the need for post-hoc military interventions to quell civil unrest. It was during these years that the United States began to act more in keeping with the classic model of imperialism—Cuban leaders were pressured to govern in ways that were amenable to North American business.

The Zayas Administration (1921–1925)

As part of its program of "prophylactic intervention" in Cuban politics, the United States dispatched Enoch Crowder to Cuba in January of 1921 as a special representative of the U.S. president. Crowder's task was to oversee partial new elections in areas that had been plagued by violence and repression during the November, 1920 voting. He was also supposed to draw up a new electoral code that would hopefully prevent such disturbances in the future. Crowder took his mission seriously, and immediately began penning a series of terse, instructive memos to President Zayas regarding the reforms he (Crowder) believed were necessary to stabilize the Cuban government and prop up the failing economy. One of the first of these recommendations involved replacing several notoriously corrupt cabinet members with individuals of Crowder's own choosing. Crowder essentially black-mailed President Zayas into accepting this dictate, by refusing to authorize a $50 million loan agreement to bail out Cuba's failed banks[4] until the so-called "honest cabinet" was installed.

After Crowder departed and the loan was secured, Zayas immediately dismissed the honest cabinet and replaced them with trusted clients. Zayas made his son, Alfredo Zayas, Jr. director of the lottery,[5] put his brother Francisco in charge of the Department of Public Instruction and later made him Minister to France, made his son-in-law comptroller-general of the republic, and his cousin Carlos Portela Secretary of the Treasury. Eventually, fourteen members of the Zayas clan found strategic and lucrative government positions in the last two years of his presidency. According to Norton (1926:82), "his forces thus distributed then laid siege to the public treasury."

Health Trends in the Zayas Regime

Public works and public health continued to suffer from this governmental instability and corruption during the Zayas regime. Records show that the first major water and sewer lines in Santiago were constructed by the American occupying army in 1901. Despite dramatic population growth throughout the early republican period, and construction of many new residential areas in the 1920s and 1930s, Santiago did not receive any additional waterworks until the 1940s, even though a $7 million dollar contract was awarded to a (politically connected) Cuban construction firm during the Zayas regime (International Bank for Reconstruction and Development, 1950). One critical USPHS official described the resulting health conditions in Santiago as follows,

Sanitary conditions in Santiago de Cuba continued during to be prominent by their absence. At various times during the year, particularly when the political campaign was at its height, the collection of garbage in the city was suspended entirely. The result was that people in all parts of the city simply threw their waste into the streets where it remained for days unless an extra heavy rain washed it to the lowlands along the water front. Since the visit of President Zayas with many prominent Americans to Santiago at the middle of December for the dedication of the Roosevelt memorial, an effort has been made to collect garbage at night from houses fronting on paved streets. As a majority of the streets of the city are not paved a considerable part of the population is still without proper garbage removal service. In many of the unpaved streets there are pools of sewage that emit terrible odors and constitute menaces of the worst kind to the public health. One severe epidemic of typhoid fever was experienced in the latter part of the summer. Later an outbreak of a malignant type of dysentery was reported. Malaria fever is prevalent everywhere in an increasing degree . . . (F.R. Stewart, Annual Report upon Commerce and Industries for 1924, Santiago-de-Cuba, January 27, 1925).

Clean water remained scarce in Cuba, but one important health achievement did take place during the Zayas regime. In the early 1920s a major smallpox vaccination campaign was undertaken, and the last recorded case of the disease in Cuba was in February of 1923 (USPHS report, undated, early 1920s). Waterborne diseases, on the other hand, remained a serious problem.

The Machado Regime (1925–1933)

Collective popular dissatisfaction with Cuba's political system led to the inauguration in 1925 of a new regime, with a new rhetoric and new formula designed to save the Cuban republic from its downward spiral. Gerardo Machado began his term of office with a specific ten-point campaign of pro-business, nationalistic legislation. This was designed to placate the disgruntled American businessmen who by this point controlled nearly all aspects of sugar production, and to offer Cubans a hope of national development and stability through increased commercial prosperity and an end to the colonial model of government based on patronage. According to one American observer:

. . . Cuba is cleaning house. Her curse for years was the professional politician. When President Machado took office and astoundingly enforced his slogan of a 'business administration' graft was rampant. Men holding sinecures were paid not on one payroll but on three or four. One chauffeur was a lieutenant of police, an officer in the navy and a collector of revenue. Machado changed all that. He has done his best to abolish petty graft. Cuba is at last getting a decent government (Woon, 1929:281).

Machado also undertook a number of major public works improvements in the late 1920s, financed in part with an $80 million loan from the Chase Manhattan Bank. Few if any of these dollars, however, were directed toward public health improvements. Havana's drinking water (and presumably that of other cities as well) remained contaminated, and the loan instead funded construction of the central highway and the extravagant national Capitol building, as well as a number of developments intended to promote tourism.

The onset of Prohibition in the United States in 1920 meant that Cuba became instantly desirable as a resort destination where alcohol could be legally enjoyed, often to great excess.[6] New hotels and casinos were constructed, and a major beautification campaign was undertaken in the city of Havana. A Chicago syndicate headed by John McEntee Bowman and Charles Flynn took control of the Havana race track and Jockey Club, subsequently branching out into real estate developments designed to make Cuba "the new playground of the Western world" (*New York Times*, February 26, 1928). Machado also liberalized divorce laws, hoping to encourage divorce tourism and divert North American business away from western cities like Las Vegas and Reno, Nevada (Phillips, 1935).

Despite Machado's promising rhetoric, his regime quickly began to resemble that of his predecessors. Graft, patronage, violence and personalism all became increasingly common through the late 1920s and early 1930s. These practices, combined with the economic disintegration that resulted from the onset of the Great Depression in the United States led to the formation of an increasingly bitter and violent opposition movement that effectively paralyzed the public sector and destroyed a good deal of Cuba's political and economic infrastructure for many years.

Health Trends in the Machado Era

USPHS reports from Havana in the 1920s include lists of reportable infectious diseases, such as typhoid, malaria, measles, smallpox and other health conditions that might spread to the United States via contaminated steamships. While the numbers cited in these reports were probably not a very accurate measure of the scope of the disease in Havana,[7] they do provide a general indicator of the extent of Havana's ongoing problems with waterborne and vector borne infections during this time period.

The two greatest infectious contributors to mortality in Havana during the 1920s were malaria and typhoid fever. Between fiscal years

TABLE 8.1
Morbidity and Mortality rates for Havana's leading causes of death
during the 1920s (source: USPHS records)

Fiscal Year	Typhoid Cases Havana	Typhoid Deaths Havana	Havana Population estimate	Mortality rate per 100,000 popluation
1921–1922	357	71	650,000	10.92
1922–1923	716	158	650,000	24.3
1923–1924	570	95	650,000	14.6
1924–1935	937	85	650,000	13.07
1925–1926	399	82	650,000	12.6
1926–1927	540	100	650,000	15.4
1928–1929	319	60	650,000	9.2
1929–1930	287	60	650,000	9.2

1921–22 and 1928–1929 there was an average of around 800 cases of malaria per year in Havana, which in turn averaged about 18 deaths. The same time period saw an average of 515 cases of typhoid fever per year, with an average of eighty-eight deaths. There was significant fluctuation in number of cases from year to year. Typhoid ranged from a high of 716 cases in 1922–1923 to a low of 287 cases in 1928–1929.

In the USPHS reports, there is little information provided about mosquito eradication programs in the Cuba during the 1920s. Given the intensity of mosquito control efforts during the U.S. military occupations of Cuba, and the near eradication of mosquito borne diseases in the city of Havana under the U.S. occupation, it seems reasonable to hypothesize that all of Cuba's *caudillo* presidents allowed these programs to lapse during the early republican era. In the case of waterborne infections such as typhoid, USPHS reports (as well as other documents) do contain a good deal of information on the sociopolitical causes of Havana's contaminated drinking water.

A USPHS report from Havana in the early 1920s described in detail the ongoing problems with the city's water supply,

Every year in May or June, the water supply of Havana becomes a serious problem. If only the Vento [spring] water is used, it is good quality but insufficient in quantity. Even in the lower part of the town there is not always enough pressure to send the water to the second floor in day time. Many people have to wait for the night and make provision for the next day's use. If the sluices of the Almendares River are opened and that water allowed to mix with that that of the Vento collecting reservoir, the quantity is sufficient, but as this is the rainy season the Almendares River is contaminated with mud, organic detritus and germs, for the Almendares flows through a district that is closely inhabited and highly cultivated. From the Vento reservoir the water goes to the Distributing Reservoir at Palatino, on a hill. Here a chlorinating plant has been established. This when properly used is said to be sufficient to destroy the germs, but as the water is not filtered, mud and organic detritus are distributed with it. . . . Naturally all this causes great discussions among all classes; studies and inspections are made. But by the end of the summer when the water is abundant again, the discussions are stopped and nothing is done, until the next year, when everything is begun again. The present Alcalde [mayor, of Havana] has asked for an appropriation of half a million dollars to solve the Havana water problem. It is sincerely hoped that something practical will be done (USPHS report from Havana, undated, early 1920s).

The "sincere hopes" of the USPHS with respect to the water supply of Havana were to be repeatedly disappointed. Despite the $500,000 appropriation requested by the city's mayor, little or nothing was done to improve the water and typhoid epidemics recurred annually in Havana throughout the 1920s. In fact, the above passage (with the exception of the final two sentences) was repeated almost verbatim in every annual USPHS report on record from Havana between 1921 and 1929.

In 1924 USPHS officers noted that a new municipal proposal had been made for improving Havana's water supply that "would take relatively short time, would not cost much and would not interfere with any future permanent improvement on a larger scale, but on the contrary would help." In fact, the report noted that a similar proposition had been presented in the Cuban House of Representatives three times previously (in 1918, 1919 and 1924), but that no action had ever been taken. The report concluded emphatically, "The scarcity of water has lasted twelve years and is getting worse. It is time something should be done." Unfortunately nothing was done, and typhoid continued to be a significant health problem.

While the USPHS was critical of the political inertia underlying Havana's ongoing water and sanitation problems, but nowhere near as critical as Cuban citizens themselves. On July 18, 1924 (in the midst of a severe typhoid epidemic) the newspaper *La Lucha* published the following vocal critique,

The only ones to blame [for the epidemic] are the inhabitants of Havana, who committed the grave error of electing a man that is absolutely worthless as an official for Mayor of Havana.[8] This is the real plague we are suffering from. If our people knew what they were about and elected competent and honest officials we would not be suffering from all the evils now have befallen us. Let us first purify the administration and afterwards our aqueducts (quoted in E.H. Crowder letter to Secretary of State, August 4, 1924).

It should be noted that Cuba's public health and sanitation departments did respond very promptly when an epidemic broke out. One USPHS report lauded the Cuban efforts to control the typhoid epidemic, "As usual in such cases [the annual epidemic of typhoid] very strict measures were taken by the sanitary authorities" (USPHS report, 1924). The Cuban Ministry of Sanitation issued water advisories throughout the city urging people to boil their drinking water, and anti-typhoid injections were made mandatory throughout the island. Additional chlorine was added at the (inadequate) water treatment plant. During one of the more severe outbreaks in 1924 the municipal departments of Public Works and Sanitation engaged in "a thorough cleaning and disinfecting of the city water works . . . [with] broken water mains mended" (Report of E.H. Crowder to Secretary of State, August 1924). These actions, however, constituted posthoc treatments that slowed the course of the epidemic, but did not prevent future outbreaks from occurring.

Health Services

It is also important to point out that despite these lapses in public health and vector control, Cuba's private sector health resources during the 1920s were relatively plentiful. Cuban presidents often invested in hospital construction as a symbol both of progressive modernity and of their own paternalistic concern for the well-being of their citizens. As early as 1927, Cuba had thirty public and seven private hospitals (Lopez del Valle, 1927). By 1933 there were an additional twenty-six private charity hospitals in Cuba (with a total of 4,529 beds)[9]. One 1935 report stated,

Medical facilities for the poor of Havana are abundant. There are over 3,000 free hospital beds, one per 180 inhabitants, and one poor relief physician for each 2,964 population. . . . The overwhelming discrepancy between the capital and the interior is not quite so great as it appears. Many of the large hospitals in the capital are supported by national funds, and great numbers of indigents come to Havana from the interior for hospitalization (Commission on Cuban Affairs, 1935:119).

At the end of the 1950s there were 97 public hospitals in Cuba (with a total of 21,141 beds) and at least twenty-six private hospitals providing an estimated 4,500 additional beds. In addition, several American corporations such as United Fruit and the mining companies in Oriente province also maintained private company hospitals and health facilities on their more remote plantations for workers and their families.

Clinical (i.e., non-hospital based) medical care during the 1920s was often provided by mutualist associations. Members paid a small monthly fee and were subsequently entitled to subsidized health care and an array of other social services. Most of these organizations were based on ethnicity and included such powerful entities as the Centro Gallego, the Centro Austuriano, as well as various labor organizations. Estimates hold that between 36–50 percent of Havana's population were covered under some form of mutualism prior to 1959 (Danielson, 1979; Diaz-Briquets, 1983). In the words of one report from 1935, "Cuba is the scene of one of the most successful experiments in the world in cooperative medicine, a service performed by a number of cooperative societies for more than a hundred thousand members" (Commission on Cuban Affairs, 1935:22).

Mutualist health care associations were actually part of a larger network of social organizations and activities directed by a number of immigrant clubs. The Centro Gallego had over 86,000 members in 1952 and an annual budget of $1.5 million. In addition to operating its own hospitals and health clinics, the center also maintained a private bank, a school, a sanitarium, private stores and foundations as well as providing pensions for retired members. The Asturian Club also had over 70,000 members in 1952 and offered a similar array of services.

The exclusively ethnic orientation of the Centro Gallego and the Centro Austuriano, of course, meant that their membership was limited to those of direct Spanish ancestry—in other words, blacks or people of color were not allowed. A number of parallel organizations were also founded that provided mutualist health services to these other social groups. In this sense, the character of pre-revolutionary health services often mirrored existing social and economic divisions. Private fee-for-service physicians (both in Havana and in the United States) served the wealthiest of the elites, while organizations like the Centro Gallego and the Centro Austuriano served the middle class as well as newly arrived Spanish immigrants. The nonwhite middle class correspondingly formed its own (usually trade-based) mutualist associations, and the urban poor were left with an (often insufficient) array of public hospitals and charitable institutions. The rural poor were often left without health facilities at all, unless they were able to journey to a major city.

These improvements in provision of health services, however, did not necessarily have a major impact as far as improving overall health conditions for the population. As previously mentioned, health is a complex phenomenon that does not correlate in a linear fashion with the expansion of clinical medicine. As a number of researchers have shown, major shifts in population health (such as the control or eradication of infectious diseases in Europe and North America) have resulted more often from environmental changes such as improvements in housing and water supplies and better living standards than from advances in clinical medicine (Barrett et al., 1998; Dubos, 1959; McKeown, 1979; Rogers and Hackenberg, 1987).

Health Decline

In Cuba, the provision of health services to the population probably helped arrest a number of epidemics, but it did not correct the environmental conditions that led to the disease outbreak in the first place. Waterborne infections remained significant contributors to mortality in many interior cities and towns throughout the 1920s. There was an epidemic of amebic dysentery in Baracoa (a town in Oriente province) in the fall of 1924, with sixty-six recorded cases and seventeen deaths (USPHS report, 1924). The city apparently had no water treatment facilities. According to the USPHS report, "a great many laundresses washed the clothes in the river above where the city took its water supply . . . " (USPHS report, 1924). Due to the poor condition of local roads and the scarcity of doctors in the area, the epidemic was much more difficult to contain than an outbreak in Havana would have been. Frequent typhoid epidemics were also recorded in Guines, Colon,

Santiago, Camaguey and many small towns throughout the 1920s (USPHS report, August 14, 1925).

Beals (1934:307) claimed that public health deteriorated tremendously under Machado and that resurgent epidemics of malaria and other diseases swept through the population. In September, 1933 Carlos Finlay told the *New York Times* that major outbreaks of malaria had resulted from the chaos and disintegration of the national government (September 3, 1933). Documents from the provincial archives in Santiago also lend support these claims. Local *alcaldes* in Oriente often wrote to petition the provincial governor to do something about the growing public health threat, describing sanitary services as being in "a complete state of abandonment" in the later years of Machado's rule.

These (private and confidential) reports of health decline and political mismanagement stand in sharp contrast to official Cuban government propaganda extolling progress and "great victories" in health and sanitation. During the Machado regime, a series of books and articles were published describing the General's personal concern for the health of the Cuban people and featuring detailed descriptions of hospital construction, charity work, and disease eradication throughout the island (Secretaria de Sanidad y Beneficia, 1931; Lopez-Silvero, 1926; 1930). One group of visiting American journalists who came to Cuba to investigate the accounts of violence, torture and resurgent epidemic disease in Cuba under Machado described how they were instead given an official tour that highlighted the General's accomplishments in public health and public works (*New York Times*, October 21, 1930).

> Thus the answer to the charge that General Machado's friends had abused the Constitution to continue him in office for another six years was to point to a gleaming new hospital; the answer to the charge that opponents of the government had been denied opportunity to organize a party was an immaculate new high school; the answer to the charge that the President has burdened the country with heavy taxation to carry out his ambitious program was a model industrial city where the workers live in better homes than they enjoy in the United States.

In fact, it appears that health deteriorated noticeably under Machado for the simple reason that the last years of his rule precipitated tremendous political violence, civil unrest and gang warfare that led to the complete destruction of most government function for about five years (Aguilar, 1972; Alvarez del Real, 1942; Beals, 1935; Philips, 1935). According to one source, Machado closed all public hospitals and destroyed records of resurgent epidemics of malaria, typhoid and parasitism during his rule. These claims are corroborated by two independent investigators of the time, one Cuban (Mencia, 1936), and one American (Commission on Cuban Affairs, 1935).

One physician from the town of Guantanamo wrote to U.S. Secretary of State Cordell Hull in October of 1933 (shortly after the fall of the Machado regime) describing the complete deterioration of health and sanitation under Machado's rule, and begging for the United States to "remember its obligations" and intervene under Article Five of the Platt Amendment to remedy the situation,

> Sanitary conditions in all the cities of the Island are a disgrace to any civilized country. The Health Department exists only in name. Malaria, which is endemic, has increased in alarming proportions. I am willing to testify before competent authorities that in the district of Guantanamo alone there are more than 500 cases of this disease. Typhoid Fever, which normally runs to about fifteen or twenty cases a year in the district, has gone up to about 150 cases. The streets of the city have not been swept in two months, and everywhere there can be found ill smelling piles of garbage with the ever-present swarm of flies. . . . Does Secretary of State Hull sincerely believe that the present problem can be settled between the Cubans? And if so, why does he not expedite the magic formula [intervention under Article Five] so that the country and four million people can be saved from death and starvation? . . . It is a matter of life and death to the inhabitants of Cuba that present conditions be changed, whether by military intervention or by setting up a Cuban as Provisional President with a cabinet worthy of the name, and BACKED BY AMERICAN TROOPS TO REESTABLISH ORDER and bring back common sense . . . (Letter from Dr. E.A. Baradat to U.S. Embassy, November 6, 1933, emphasis in original).

The Decline of Cuba Libre

Epidemic infectious disease was not the only unfortunate consequence of Cuba's *caudillo* governments during the Platt era. Public education also suffered greatly from Cuba's cycles of violence and instability during this time. During the War of Independence in 1899, illiteracy in Cuba was estimated to be approximately sixty-five percent. Education thus became one of the chief priorities of the U.S. provisional administration under Leonard Wood. In June 1900, under the American occupation, school enrollment increased almost tenfold to 143,000. This expansion of education was financed entirely through Cuban customs revenues, not direct taxation. Additional American funds were spent by the U.S. to train Cuban teachers, a number of whom were sent to a special training program at Harvard.

The Estrada Palma administration tried to maintain this investment in education, and in 1902 his budget allotted $15 million, or one fourth of the national budget to education, with an average enrollment of seventy-two pupils for each 1,000 inhabitants. The Department of Education under Estrada Palma had 3,600 employees (Beals, 1934; Norton, 1926). By 1911 school enrollment had declined to forty-nine per 1,000 inhabitants (Lockmiller, 1938:135), yet department of education payroll had *increased* to support 6,000 employees. Despite this vast expansion of the government's education payroll, enrollment, matriculation, and literacy rates continued to decline—illiteracy among white youths increased 15 percent, and among people of color, 25 percent (Norton, 1926:81).

A final note must be added about costs of all this graft and patronage to Cuban citizens. In 1910, Irene Wright (p. 160) stated that the Cuban government was, "the most expensive government on earth" and that, "those who operate it (the Cuban office-holding class) have every reason to labor to make it even more so, since its extravagances run to salaries, which they receive . . . " For most of the Platt era, almost 85 percent of all government funds were generated from customs revenues, which were steadily increased to support the growing extravagance of the state. Given that Cuba imported nearly all of its basic foodstuffs (51 percent of all imports were food and clothing— essential, not luxuries), this amounted to a massive form of hidden taxation, leveled equally upon the wealthy as the poor, for all basic necessities of life.

In 1909, total customs duties in Cuba amounted to approximately $12 per capita. In comparison, customs dues in the U.S. were only $3.55 per capita (figures cited in Wright, 1910:198). Wright goes on to state, "these other countries maintain the tariff fence at their ports to protect . . . home industries of their own, Cuba maintains hers frankly for the sole purpose of getting cash to keep her government, for she has no industries to protect." By 1926 Cuban citizens paid between

$30 and $45 million per year, or about $10 to $15 per capita in customs dues, three or four times higher than the United States at this time (Norton, 1926).

Furthermore, in the 1920s Cubans were also assessed another $10 per capita in internal taxes. Lottery revenues amounted to another $12 million diverted from citizens to the state coffers. All in all, it was estimated that the official cost of supporting the Cuban government amounted to approximately $25–40 per capita, plus many additional unofficial payments for, "little extortions and petty tributes which [a Cuban] must pay every time he comes in contact with an official but which never show in the accounts" (Norton, 1926:84). In comparison, the cost per capital of government in Puerto Rico was only $11, and provided (in the words of one observer), "all the blessings of good government, protection of life and property, schools, roads, libraries and many other things of which the Cuban does not even dream" (Norton, 1926).

Many noted Cuban intellectuals observing these trends penned sharp critiques of national politics during the 1920s, frequently describing a subjective sense of decline and regression in health, education and overall national development due to these cycles of political corruption, violence and instability (Fernandez, 1916; Ortiz, 1924; Roig, 1925). In 1924, Fernando Ortiz wrote a pamphlet entitled "La Decadencía Cubana" in which he stated, "Our homeland is facing a tremendous crisis. It is not a crisis of government, nor a crisis of a [political] party, nor a crisis of class, it is a crisis of the whole community . . . Cuban society is falling apart . . . Cuba is falling rapidly into barbarism. . . . We don't progress . . . we are falling backwards and losing our civilization."

These sentiments reflect the frustrated nationalism of Cuba's genuine patriots, who for a generation had been forced to watch as a series of avaricious political leaders had drained the country's resources and accumulated great personal wealth, but had accomplished little or nothing in the way of national "development" for Cuba. There is no doubting the resonance of this message of loss and betrayal among the Cuban populace, but the non-electoral nature of Cuban political succession combined with the *caudillos*' collective monopoly on violence effectively relegated these individuals to the sidelines of political participation.

Notes

1. The USPHS records at the National Archives in College Park, Maryland contain annual reports from the Havana office for the 1920s, but there are no records from 1909-1920.
2. The local term for this practics was "*botellas*," baby-bottles that were used to feed public officials.
3. Some historical documentation is in order to support this statement. Cuba's first president, Tomás Estrada Palma was exiled for his political activities against Spain in the late 1800s. Estrada Palma is unique in Cuban history in that after he was deposed from power he did not attempt to re-take the presidency by force and instead retired to an ancestral farm in Bayamo. Estrada Palma's successor, José Miguel Gómez went into exile after losing the 1905 election. During his exile he helped organize the "revolution" of 1906 that eventually put him in power. After his term of office, Gómez attempted to return to power in the 1917 insurrection. This attempt failed and he was imprisoned briefly before being allowed to escape into exile in Miami. Gómez' successor, Mario Menocal successfully held on to power for two terms, then was deposed in the violent 1921 elections. Menocal went into exile in Miami, then unsuccessfully attempted to return to power in a 1931 insurrection against Machado, after which he was briefly imprisoned. Menocal's successor, Alfredo Zayas narrowly escaped imprisonment by hiding out in a friend's country estate following the insurrection of 1917. Zayas' successor, Gerardo Machado imprisoned nearly all of his political enemies during the last years of his term. Machado's opposition retaliated by assassinating and violently looting the homes of Machado supporters once they obtained power in the "revolution" of 1933. The details of Fidel Castro's imprisonment during the Batista years are well known.
4. It should be noted that the Banco Nacional de Cuba (at the time, the most important financial institution on the island with over 121 branches) failed in part because of massive bank fraud perpetrated by its leaders, both of whom were close associates of President Menocal. When the scandal was discovered, one bank director committed suicide and the other fled to Europe. Over $9 million had been misappropriated. For details of these events see Jenks, 1929.
5. The Cuban national lottery was a major source of graft and patronage throughout the twentieth century.
6. One enthusiastic guidebook writer in 1929 noted that even the Havana jail maintained "a first class bar contiguous to the guest chamber" (Woon, 1929:6).
7. The USPHS officers who wrote the reports were careful to point out a number of factors interfered with accurate data collection. These included the tendency of poor patients to avoid the formal health care system for lack of funds, the tendency for health professionals to underreport mild cases of disease, as well as the tendency for sick individuals to travel from the provinces to Havana to seek medical treatment. The mortality rates cited were described as accurate, since they were taken from mortuary records.

8. The position of Mayor of Havana was considered the second most profitable political job on the island, second only to the Presidency in terms of graft opportunities.
9. These developments have frequently been overlooked by contemporary scholars. De Brun and Elling (1987:688), for instance, claimed erroneously that in 1959 there was only "one rural hospital" in Cuba.

9

Health and Disease in the Gangster State, 1934–1959

Havana has always maintained lucrative vice and smuggling trades, even during the colonial era (Robert, 1953; López Levia, 1930; Schwartz, 1989; Suchlicki, 1997). The development of international tourism in the 1920s greatly expanded Cuba's vice markets, and foreign tourists eagerly partook of all of Havana's forbidden pleasures: prostitution, pornography, alcohol, tobacco and narcotic drugs. The seamier side of the city was described quite colorfully by one guidebook writer from the 1920s,

> The triangular pocket nearest the wharves is a prurient spot resorted to by courtezans varying in complexion . . . who unblushingly loll about heavy-eyed and languorous in abbreviated and diaphanous costumes, nictitating with incendiary eyes at passing masculinity; studiously displaying their physical charms or luring the stranger by flaming words or maliciously imperious gestures. These gossamer wantons with loving dispositions . . . here practice the scarlet arts of aphasia and sacrifice themselves upon the altar of Aphrodite. As a rule they appeal only to the hedonist callous to moral degradation or to the lethal consequences of malignantly poisonous diseases (Terry, 1929: 200).

Early in the 1920s, bootleggers from the United States found Cuba to be an ideal smuggling center and formed lucrative partnerships with Cuban politicians to expand their trade. Al Capone constructed a lavish house on Varadero Beach, and Charles "Lucky" Luciano and Meyer Lansky traveled frequently to Cuba on business as well. In some cases alcohol purchased in Europe was offloaded in Cuba, then smuggled by boat into the United States. In other cases, bootleggers contracted with Cuban distilleries to produce rum for export to dry northern cities (*New York Times*, April 28, 1929).

It is a standard rule of smuggling that once an illicit pipeline has been successfully established between two countries, it will naturally expand to include all manner of contraband. By the late 1920s, underground networks originally developed to smuggle alcohol had developed into vast international criminal syndicates transporting narcotics, weapons and illegal immigrants between the United States, Mexico, Canada and Cuba.

In 1929 hundreds of pounds of opium were seized in Cuba in a single raid that resulted in the arrest of several members of the Cuban customs police and the army (*New York Times*, April 23, 1929). In January 1931 a raid on another Havana den netted sixty pounds of opium, along with "large quantities" of cocaine and other narcotic drugs (*New York Times*, January 25, 1931). These seizures most likely represented only a small percentage of the actual flow of drugs and contraband passing through the country.

In 1926 the growing influence of these syndicates so concerned North American authorities that a new treaty was negotiated between Washington, DC and Havana "to prevent the illegal entry into or departure from the shores of either country of aliens and also the smuggling of articles of all kinds, particularly narcotics" (*New York Times*, March 12, 1926). The treaty was unsuccessful, and subsequent newspaper reports indicated that the traffic in contraband (and illegal aliens) from Cuba to the United States continued to increase.

During this time, political office in Cuba became even more economically valuable than it had been under previous administrations because of the informal taxes that could be levied on smuggling revenues. A form of mutualism evolved, with favored criminals granted lucrative concessions in the underground economy in return for providing political leaders with a significant percentage of their earnings.[1] Working together in this way allowed gangsters and politicians to establish a collective monopoly on vice. By 1924 these arrangements had become so lucrative that seats in the Cuban senate were openly bought and sold as investment commodities. For fifteen to twenty thousand dollars, an aspiring politician could purchase a political office, and then use the power of that office to recoup the investment losses and gain a substantial profit through various forms of political extortion (detailed in the *New York Times*, March 29th, 1924).

These criticisms should not be taken to imply that the United States was free of corruption during this era. To the contrary, the decade of the 1920s was one of the most corrupt in American history. Bootleggers freely sold contraband alcohol to judges, policemen, and society matrons throughout the United States. Individual policemen were paid huge sums by racketeers to guard liquor shipments or to selectively arrest unwanted competitors. In the public sector, indigenous "graft cliques" like New York's Tammany Hall were operating in most major cities. Even Enoch Crowder (who so fiercely criticized the Zayas administration for its corruption) described a pronounced sense of shame when he returned home to Chicago and witnessed the violence and corruption associated with municipal politics in his own city (detailed in Guggenheim, 1934).

There were, however, some key structural difference between the way North American and Cuban political corruption were configured that resulted in the creation of a different political-economic forms in Cuba. In the United States, aspiring gangsters could purchase "protection" from authorities in something of a free market system. While rival gangsters might try to limit entrepreneurship in vice markets, political officials did not. The police and army in the United States might have tolerated smuggling (for a price) but they did not use their arms and training to establish and defend economic monopolies for favored gangsters. In Cuba, however, *caudillos* sought exclusive government control over economic activities in the informal economy and established their own personalistic, armed groups to protect this lucrative economic territory. As a result, organized crime groups became fused with the formal political sector in Cuba in ways that they were not in the United States.

After Prohibition, it is misleading to speak of "organized crime" as separate or distinct from "politics" in Cuba. Instead, activities in the illicit economy often configured events in the formal political sector, and vice versa. Cuba became literally a gangster-state, and it was often difficult to find a clear dividing line between the world of organized crime and the world of Cuban politics. As one newspaper editorial stated in 1931, "Cuba is as gang-ridden as . . . Chicago, with this difference: Cuba's gangsters wear the mask of government while those of Chicago do not" (quoted in Cuban Information Bureau, 1931).

These dynamics are clearly visible in the events surrounding the overthrow of Machado in 1933. Despite compelling humanitarian rhetoric, once in power these revolutionaries immediately began fighting with one another over the spoils of office, as well as contracting with North American criminal syndicates to further enrich themselves by expanding Havana's gambling, smuggling and vice industries.

The Revolution of 1933

In 1930 the onset of the Great Depression in the United States plunged the Cuban economy into chaos, and left many workers and their families facing near starvation. City laborers saw their wages fall from $3.00 to .50 per day, and rural wages fell from approximately $1.50 to .25 per day (Hoernel, 1976). This economic crisis greatly intensified popular dissatisfaction, and further unified the Machado opposition. With the formal sector of the economy practically destroyed, political office was viewed as one of the few guaranteed means of earning substantial income in Cuba, and the anti-Machado opposition correspondingly intensified.

Machado responded to attacks on his rule with increasing violence, and turned loose all the forces of the state (police, soldiers and a special terrorist squad known as the "Porra") loose upon the citizenry to suppress the broad-based opposition movement. The radical student groups and opposition *caudillo*s in turn contracted with North American criminal syndicates to arm themselves for the increasingly violent struggle against Machado. Contraband was taken out of Cuba, and arms, ammunition and explosives were smuggled in (Ambassador Henry Guggenheim, report to U.S. State Department, undated; Lumen, 1935). The gangsters themselves were essentially exploiting both sides of this conflict, smuggling contraband for Machado and his henchmen as well as providing arms to the students in order to secure favorable concessions for themselves in the event the opposition was successful in taking power.

By 1931 the anti-Machado movement had escalated practically to a state of civil war, leading one author to state, "terror had become the principal means of government" (Levine, 1993). Since many of the young students arrayed against Machado were from Havana's leading families, the state's policy of torture and murder for opposition leaders was especially explosive. The violence left no one untouched, and politicized many of Havana's elite families who had previously sought to remain neutral. The direction of this politicization was more often occasioned by personal vendettas than by political ideology.

Increasingly bitter opposition groups began to target all Machado followers, or anyone affiliated with the national government for assassination. Often these were vengeance killings, designed to retaliate against the repeated torture-murders perpetrated by Machado's secret police. Frequent and protracted strikes carried out by various labor groups under control of the Communist Party paralyzed vast sections of the economy, resulting in tremendous inflation of food prices and paralysis of commerce.

Both sides of the conflict again tried to force the United States into the fray on their behalf. The Machado opposition groups maintained a powerful exile junta that aggressively lobbied U.S. statesmen and newspapers with propaganda about their plight—gaining much sympathy from prominent leftists such as journalist Carleton Beals[2]. Machado himself clung to his pro-business credentials and tried to use his contacts with American capitalists to influence U.S. foreign policy. A key issue was an $80 million short-term loan that Machado had obtained from the Chase Manhattan Bank. Machado insinuated to the bankers that if he were deposed and the opposition allowed to take power, they would declare that the loan had been illegally contracted and refuse to honor the repayment terms (as has happened when Menocal took power after the revolution of 1912 and refused to repay loans brokered by the Gómez administration). Thus the U.S. state department was besieged by all sides to intervene in Cuba—both to overthrow and to support Gerardo Machado. As pressure to intervene intensified, the U.S. State Department finally sent Sumner Welles to try and negotiate a solution to Cuba's escalating conflicts in May of 1933.

Welles arrived in Havana in the midst of deepening violence. His early dispatches to Washington, DC describe shootouts, riots and labor strikes, with sometimes as many as twelve bombs exploding in Havana in a single day. During this time the *New York Times* reported "complete anarchy" in the interior cities and towns (September 24, 1933). After much diplomatic maneuvering Welles finally managed to broker Machado's resignation. Immediately upon Machado's departure, homes and officers of Machado supporters throughout the country were targeted for looting, and armed student gangs began to seize control of government offices at gunpoint. Several Machado policemen who did not flee the country were hunted down by angry mobs and murdered on the streets of Havana, their bodies left hanging from street lamps as a warning against other Machado followers foolish enough to remain in Cuba (Phillips, 1935).

To try and control the growing anarchy, Welles installed the moderate Carlos Manuel de Cespedes as President. Cespedes, however, was not accepted by the majority of student radicals, and his regime was quickly overthrown in favor of a coalition led by University of Havana professor Ramón Grau San Martín. Soon after the revolt against Cespedes, the enlisted men in the army added to the national chaos by staging a rebellion against their "Machadista" officers. The officer corps took refuge in the opulent Hotel Nacional. A tense standoff ensued for several weeks, and eventually fighting broke out. The hotel was shelled for several days until a truce could be brokered. The leader of the Sergeant's revolt, Fulgencio Batista, would go on to maintain personal control over army in Cuba until the Castro revolution in 1959.

Grau San Martín and the Pentarchy

Ramón Grau San Martín's first presidential administration lasted about one hundred days.[3] During this time, he did not govern alone but was part of a pentarchy that included Guillermo Portela (another professor from the University of Havana), Porfirio Franca Alvarez de la Campa (a well-known banker), Sergio Carbo (a radical journalist), and Jose Irisarri (a lawyer). In his short tenure as president Grau and the Pentarchy passed an array of legislation designed to ease Cuba's economic crisis and improve social and economic conditions for workers. Grau supervised the abrogation of the Platt Amendment, decreed an eight hour day, created a department of labor, reduced electricity rates by forty percent, prohibited the importation of illegal workers from Haiti and Jamaica, passed a law forcing all employers to hire at least a 50 percent Cuban workforce, gave women the right to vote, and proposed land reform.

Grau also passed legislation making the University of Havana an autonomous territory. The radical student opposition groups (his key supporters) had suffered terribly at the hands of Machado, and this step was intended to prevent any future government from engaging in such brutal repression against students. From 1933 on, no national police or army were allowed to set foot on the campus, which elected its own government and police force[4] (Aguilar, 1972; Thomas, 1998; Langley, 1989; Suchlicki, 1969).

In most conventional narratives of Cuba's twentieth century history, Grau's radical nationalist legislation is described as threatening to the North American capitalists and wealthy landowners who controlled Cuba's economy. The subsequent refusal of the United States to recognize the Grau administration is portrayed as the key factor in configuring its downfall (Blackburn, 1963; Gott, 2004; Huberman and Sweezy, 1960; Paterson, 1994; Wright, 2001). While there is truth to this argument, it should also be noted that the radical left in Cuba was much more violently opposed to the Grau regime than the United States.

From 1928–1935 the international communist movement maintained a strictly isolationist position, attacking moderate leftists and anarchists as enemies and "tools of imperialism" who would delay the formation of a truly revolutionary worker's state. The Cuban Communist Party correspondingly denounced Grau as a reactionary leader of a "bourgeois-landlord government." In one communiqué from the Cuban Communist Party to their comrades in the United States, the Grau regime was denounced as a form of "terror unleashed against the working masses" that was "without precedent in the bloody history of the bourgeois-landlord colonial regime" (Letter from Central Committee of Cuban Communist Party to Central Committee of the United States Communist Party, reprinted in *The Daily Worker*, November 22, 1933). The Communists, using their control over Cuban labor unions, subsequently embarked on a calculated campaign to destabilizing the Grau regime through strikes and terrorism. Ironically, while the communists denounced Grau as a "reactionary executioner," Sumner Welles described him as "frankly communistic" to superiors in Washington, DC (detailed in Aguilar, 1972; Blackburn, 1963; Alexander, 1969:273; Paterson, 1994).

Batista and Guiteras

When the first Grau regime collapsed due to the combined opposition of the United States and the radical left (as well as its own internal factionalism), the resulting power vacuum led to a period of intense instability. There were seven different Presidents in Cuba between 1933 and 1940, each one ultimately toppled by some combination of opposition from the radical left, the military, the right, various nonaligned *caudillo*s and pressure from the United States government.

The Communist Party took advantage of the confusion to try and seize control of the revolution of 1933 for itself and the Soviet Union. These efforts were surprisingly successful. By October of 1933 Soviet propaganda organs such as the *Kommunisticheski Internatsional* (Communist International) were giving the Cuban communists exclusive credit for the success of the revolution against Machado. In one dispatch it was stated, "Machado was overthrown purely by the revolutionary onslaught of the toiling masses . . . This movement has been prepared by all the preceding activities of the Communist Party of Cuba, and it was led by the Party on the whole" (quoted in letter from Felix Cole, U.S. Charge D'Affaires Havana to Secretary of State, October 13, 1933).

Under the leadership of Fabio Grobart and a number of veteran Eastern European Communist organizers, several massive sugar mills in the interior of the country were taken over by workers and declared to be "Soviet." The most notable of these were the American Sugar Refining Company's plants at Jarnou and Senado (*New York Times*, October 18, 1933). In August of 1933, the communists even attempted to organize a massive march on the Presidential Palace in Havana to install a "proletarian president" (*New York Times*, August 24, 1933). These efforts failed, but the Party did succeed in establishing itself as an important player in Cuban politics (particularly in Oriente province) for the remainder of the twentieth century. By 1939 unofficial estimates placed Party membership in Cuba between 30,000 and 50,000 individuals—a dramatic increase from the 4,000–5,000 known members of the early 1930s (Confidential Report to Secretary of State from U.S. Embassy, Havana, March 15, 1939).

Throughout all of this turmoil, Fulgencio Batista (who had promoted himself to Colonel) continued to consolidate power over the army. One of the key obstacles in Batista's move to control the government was Antonio Guiteras, Grau San Martín's radical leftist vice-president. Many of the student groups distrusted Batista and the army, and chose to remain instead under the leadership of Guiteras. To challenge Batista's forces, Grau created an independent student-based militia force known as the "Revolutionary Guard."

The leftist Revolutionary Guard often clashed with Batista's army, as well as with the militants in the communist party throughout the early 1930s, leading one Cuban newspaper to declare, "We are in open civil war," (quoted in the *New York Times*, September 21, 1933). Six people were killed in a gun battle between the army and communist party militants in the fall of 1933, and in early November over 100 Cubans were killed, and 500 taken prisoner in a battle at the Atares Castle between dissident revolutionary groups opposed to Grau (reported in the *New York Times*, November 19, 1933). A radical branch of the ABC (the secret political/terrorist organization originally formed to overthrow Machado) formally withdrew its support for Grau in October of 1933, and declared open warfare on the regular (non-radical) ABC, North American property holders and all other Grau supporters.

When Grau resigned and went into exile in early 1934, many observers fully expected Antonio Guiteras and the radical left to take control of Cuba rather than Fulgencio Batista and the army. These dynamics were described in a November, 1933 dispatch sent by Sumner Welles to the State Department in Washington, DC,

> Dr. Antonio Guiteras, the Communist Secretary of Gobernación made his resignation effective this morning. He gave it as his opinion that the failure of the [Grau] Government was due to the fact that it did not turn sharply to the left, and announced his intention of working for a government composed of soldiers, sailors, small shopkeepers and workers. He made evident a definite break between himself and Batista, because Batista was resolutely opposed to communism and the disorders promoted by labor agitators, and threatened to get rid of Batista in the near future.

Batista, however, continued to assert his power and expanded the size and scope of the army to challenge Guiteras. In January 1934, shortly after Grau's resignation, Batista used the army to disarm the police (who were often loyal to Guiteras) and take over a number of municipal functions in Oriente province. Several months later the army took control of the city of Santiago during a small uprising (*New York Times*, June 17, 1934). Guiteras continued to build support in the navy and police forces. According to the *New York Times*, by early 1934 Guiteras had control of "the entire navy, the police force and part of the army" (January 16, 1934).

The tension continued to build, and one *New York Times* reporter speculated that, "there may be a war, the navy and police [supporting

Guiteras and Grau] on one side, the army [supporting Batista] on the other" (Phillips, 1959:144). The standoff between Batista and Guiteras was finally resolved in May of 1935 when the army assassinated Guiteras at his hideout in Matanzas[5]. Batista was then able to consolidate his hold over the armed forces, and used that power as the base for his eventual takeover of the Cuban government.[6]

Radical Factions and Political Gangsters

Guiteras' radical student followers (including the revolutionary army) did not surrender or disband after the death of their leader. Many of them continued to fight against Batista in newly organized student gangs and militias. The Auténtico Party (meaning the "authentic" revolutionary party, as opposed to Batista's movement) was founded by Grau and his followers in 1934 to carry on this struggle. The Auténticos tried to unite some of the leftist groups and student activists into a single force, but fragmentation and factionalism remained a problem. By 1935 the radical left in Cuba had splintered into at least ten bitterly opposed groups,[7] many of which engaged in widespread violence, extortion and racketeering to finance their political struggles (Lumen, 1934; Phillips, 1949; Thomas, 1998; Suchlicki, 1969). One report released soon after the downfall of Machado described the demoralizing effect these developments had on the young revolutionaries,

> During the past year many of the energies unleashed by the revolution [of 1933] have been frittered away; revolutionary forces once united for the purpose of overthrowing Machado are now divided against each other; few of the fine projects outlined in party manifestos have been carried into effect; the country has entered on a new period of disillusionment, if not pessimism (Commission on Cuban Affairs, 1935:1).

One of the more active and violent of the student militia groups was the ARG (Acción Revolutionaria Guiteras), founded by members of Guiteras' original group Joven Cuba. Other groups included the MSR (Movimiento Revolucionario Socialista, which also originated with Guiteras' Joven Cuba), the UIR (Union Revolucionario Insurrectional),[8] El Bonche, the DRE (Directorio Revolucionario Estudiantil, originally formed in 1927 to organize students against Machado), and the FEU (Federación de Estudiantes Universitarias) (Stokes, 1964; Thomas, 1998).

By the mid-1930s, the Soviet Union ended its extreme isolationism and shifted to a "popular front" approach that emphasized forming coalitions with a range of moderate leftist groups, and with capitalist nations. This brought the Party closer to the mainstream of Cuban politics. By 1943 the Cuban communist party (under its new name of Popular Socialist Party) was estimated to have at least 122,000 registered members. During these years the Soviet embassy often threw lavish parties and receptions in Havana that were attended by many of socially prominent (and decidedly noncommunist) elites. Many young student leaders received military training and support from the Soviet Union and a number of highly influential student leaders left Cuba for Spain to fight on the loyalist side. Others fled to Mexico to avoid persecution from Batista. Often these groups became united in exile, and some of them eventually coalesced into the Caribbean Legion—an international leftist militia composed of Cuban (and other) student radicals, Spanish Civil War veterans and young communist party members. The Legion specifically targeted Latin dictators such as Trujillo and Somoza for assassination, and tried to organize popular revolts in Venezuela, Guatemala, Nicaragua and the Dominican Republic (see Ameringer, 1996)

Batista in Power, 1934–1944

From 1934 until the Castro revolution in 1959, political power in Cuba alternated between military leader Fulgencio Batista and anti-Machado revolutionaries Grau San Martín and Carlos Prio Socarras. It is tempting to describe these political groups in terms of the "left" (Grau and the radical students) and the "right" (Batista and the army), but the situation was much more complex and defies simplistic dichotomies. Batista, for instance, originally interpreted the sergeant's rebellion he organized against the Machado officers from a leftist point of view. The violent and corrupt officer corps was understood as a tool of the Machado dictatorship, which itself was viewed as a product of capitalist corruption and imperialist exploitation. Sergeants and enlisted men, on the other hand, were understood as something of a military proletariat to be "liberated" by the revolution. Shortly after taking power Batista gave an interview to the *New York Times* in which he described himself as a "progressive socialist" and "anti-imperialist" (July 5, 1936; see also Montaner, 1981). Many of Guiteras' radical followers, on the other hand, went on to identify with the Spanish Falangist movement (a fascist organization) while others remained sympathetic to the Cuban communist party (*New York Times*, April 20, 1939).

Batista also followed something of a leftist agenda during his early years in power. He socialized a number of public services, invested in health programs and enacted land reform. In 1937 he legalized the communist party in Cuba, and appointed two leading communists to cabinet positions. These actions made the Cuban communist party the first in the hemisphere to obtain national prominence, and Cuba quickly became a base of operations for Soviet activity throughout Latin America and the Caribbean (Alexander, 1969).

Once legitimized by Batista, the communist party was able to make great inroads in consolidating its power in Cuba. In 1939 the communists won six seats in the constitutional convention, and many of the trade unions came under party control. Batista facilitated these developments, supervising the formation of the confederation of Cuban labor, which remained in the hands of the Party until the late 1940s. Despite Batista's support, a number of Cuba's communist party leaders also maintained covert alliances with the Grau and Prio backed anti-Batista underground.

In December 1940, Batista was formally elected president on a socialist-democratic platform. Six people were killed and forty wounded in election day violence (*New York Times*, July 15, 1940). The communist party's strategic alliance with Batista paid off during this time as well—Party members won over one hundred city council seats across Cuba, and communist mayors were elected in the towns of Santiago and Manzanillo (Alexander, 1968).

The Gangster-State, Part 1

While Batista followed a moderate leftist mandate during his early years in power in the 1930s, he also acted much like a traditional Cuban *caudillo*. Since the revolution of 1933 had banished Machado's officer corps as well as the dictator himself, Batista was in an ideal position to shore up his power base by building up an entirely new army under his personal control. By 1936, over one-fifth of the national budget was devoted to military expenditures. According to one scholar this was "a proportion unheard of even at the height of Machado's dictatorship" (Langley, 1989:134).

In keeping with the pattern established by earlier Cuban *caudillos*, Batista used this expanded army to seize control of more and more sectors of the national economy. In a key move designed to further disenfranchise members of Grau's (and Guiteras') rival militias (who tended to predominate in the national police force), Batista had the Cuban cabinet grant the army police powers in all cities and rural districts in Cuba (*New York Times* April 1, 1936). The military also thwarted at least one Auténtico uprising, and suppressed a counter-revolution organized by the deposed Machado officer corps (detailed in the *New York Times*, July 5, 1936 and July 9, 1936). By the late 1930s almost all secondary education, the national lottery, gambling concessions, and even much of the police force, had been placed in the hands of Batista's army. The *New York Times* expressed concern about these practices in an editorial dated May 25, 1936,

> Military authorities [in Cuba] wrested power from nearly every branch of the government and their encroachment upon civil affairs caused much dissatisfaction. The police, formerly under the Department of Interior, were incorporated into the army; into military reserve corps thousands of public employees were inducted, and recently soldiers were granted police authority in every district of the republic. The army boasts that more than 700 schools, whose teachers are members of the army, have been established; and the administration of state charity was in a large measure turned over to military authorities by recent decrees.

Batista also used his control over the military to dominate the lucrative commerce of the informal economy, and formed a close alliances with U.S. criminal syndicates to expand vice and smuggling on the island. Soon after he seized power, Batista reorganized gambling activities and placed Meyer Lansky in charge of Havana's Oriental Park racetrack as well as several national casinos. By 1940 Lansky had expanded the syndicate's holdings considerably with investments in tourism and hotels. Batista also made an arrangement with U.S. mafia chief Frank Costello that resulted in a presidential decree legalizing slot machines in 1937. By the early 1940s, Cuba was well on its way to becoming a major international vice center. One report commissioned by the U.S. narcotics bureau during this time stated, "As a result of the inefficiency and corruption in the national police system . . . all the known vices of modern civilization have prospered in Cuba for many years . . . these include murder, gambling, prostitution, and an extensive traffic in narcotics and marijuana" (quoted in Rovner, 2004).

Medicinal alcohol had remained legal in the United States during Prohibition and diversion of pharmaceutical stocks was a common tactic used by racketeers to obtain alcohol. In the case of Cuba, it appears this practice was successfully adapted to include narcotic drugs as well. By 1944 (the end of Batista's first term of office) an article in *Bohemia* noted that Cuba was importing ten times more legal and medicinal narcotics than comparable nations, and concluded, "the drug traffic in our country grows daily more alarming" (reported in the *New York Times*, October 15, 1944). A letter from U.S. narcotics agent Ray Olivera to his superiors in Washington, DC also notes that high-ranking officials in Cuba's Ministry of Health were involved in diverting legal pharmaceutical drugs to North American and Canadian organized crime syndicates (U.S. Narcotics Bureau report on narcotics trafficking in Havana, March 1947 and Ray Olivera, letter to Garland Williams, March 21, 1947). This development is key in that it reveals the deep interrelationship between formal politics and organized crime that evolved in Cuba following the overthrow of Machado. With the Minister of Health involved in large scale narcotics smuggling, it also stands to reason that less attention was paid to infectious disease control.

Health Trends Under Batista

In the area of health and sanitation, developments during Batista's first term as president appear mixed. On the one hand, Batista's early socialist orientation led to a number of reforms that most likely had positive effects on health. Santiago finally received a new water and sewer system in 1940 (the first since the American occupation in 1901), and internal public health surveillance reports[9] of the time appear much more comprehensive and detailed than from the previous era (Ortega, 1940). These reports also reveal rates of typhoid and diphtheria that appear very low in comparison with neighboring countries. In one internal sanitation report Santiago reported only 47 deaths from typhoid in 1939. This dropped down to only five after the new waterworks were constructed in 1940 (Ortega, 1940). Three deaths from diphtheria were recorded in Santiago in 1936, and only one in 1939 (Ortega, 1940).

Eighteen new hospitals were also constructed during the Batista era, including a nationwide series of maternal-infant health centers called "La ONDI" (Organización Nacional de Dispensarios Infantiles) (Statistical Abstract of the United States, 1962). In 1946 journalist Erna Fergusson reported being led on a tour of an elaborate tuberculosis sanitarium designed to showcase the progressive health programs of the Batista regime,

> Money raised by the sale of TB seals and the lottery bought the land and erected eight floors of a stupendous building that stares blindly out of thousands of windows not yet glazed, provided with huge underground heating, washing and cooking equipment not yet placed or connected. One is proudly conducted through miles of unfloored space, across great lounges and game rooms, operating theaters, and corridors of windows . . . I was assured that this is in accordance with the best Swiss theory (Fergusson, 1946:131).

In keeping with the personalistic tradition of Cuban politics, however, this extravagant sanitarium was deliberately neglected by officials of the succeeding Auténtico regimes. Fergusson concluded her report by stating, "Nothing is finished, nor is any money in sight for competition now that President Batista has been succeeded by President Grau San Martin" (1946:131).

There were also continued reports of graft, mismanagement and neglect of basic health programs in other cities and towns during the first Batista regime. In 1940 the sanitary commissioner of Manzanillo (a town in Oriente province) wrote to the provincial governor stating, "The city is in a total state of abandonment by the [sanitary] authorities. Dirt, garbage and mosquitoes now constitute an imminent danger for the inhabitants of the town." The corruption of the health sector at the national level (including the wholesale diversion of medicinal narcotics to U.S. organized crime groups) most likely had negative effects on health as well, though the lack of reliable health statistics from this time makes it difficult to draw definitive conclusions. Mortality figures cited by Diaz-Briquets (1983) also show a gradual but constant decline in deaths from infectious and parasitic disease in Cuba following the 1933 revolution, implying that living standards continued to improve, and these lapses in public health infrastructure did not have catastrophic effects on overall population health trends.

The Auténtico Era, 1944–1952

In 1944 Batista was voted out of office by his chief rival, Ramón Grau San Martín of the Auténtico Party. Like all Cuban elections, the 1944 election involved gunfire and casualties. At least two people were killed in election day violence, and many more wounded in shootouts between rival political gangs (*New York Times* October 15, 1944). According to the *New York Times*, a number of army generals under Batista were "angered by the failure of the President to use the military authorities to sway the elections for the government coalition" and began immediately plotting to assassinate Grau in order to retain their power in the military (*New York Times* June 6, 1944).

Grau responded to these threats by purging and briefly imprisoning many of Batista's military leaders. Within a month of the election, Grau had dismissed 187 of Batista's officers. Batista himself took refuge in Daytona Beach during Grau's first term of office to escape reprisals. These deposed generals subsequently fled to Mexico and began plotting a coup. Since many of the remaining soldiers were still loyal to Batista, Grau armed over 5,000 university students to act as his personal militia during his term of office (*New York Times*, November 23, 1944).

Grau's aggressive purge of Batista's army was in part due to his desire to gain control over Havana's lucrative vice markets. Despite his leftist ideology and progressive rhetoric, Grau's presidency (and that of his successor, Carlos Prio Socarras—also of the Auténtico Party) was hardly revolutionary[10]. In fact, it was marked by similar patterns of graft, corruption and violence as earlier Cuban rulers. As Langely (1989:180) has described,

> Ensconced in power, the revolutionaries of 1933 looked more and more like the grafters of the Zayas era. Batista had gotten rich in office, but Grau and his cronies stole more than he. The stench of corruption in the Cuban government during these years mas mitigated only slightly by the sweetness of sugar profits. Graft pervaded every level and was so deeply entrenched, one historian of Cuba has written, that only a thorough revolutionary cleansing could have eradicated it.

The Gangster-State, Part 2

In 1946, Tampa mafiosi Santos Trafficante Jr. took up residence in Havana to supervise a major expansion of organized crime, and to organize a powerful new narcotics smuggling syndicate. Trafficante's presence coincided with Lucky Luciano's arrival in the fall of 1946 following deportation from the United States. Soon after Luciano took up residence in Cuba, a high-level conference was convened at the Hotel Nacional to organize the expansion of the international narcotics trade. Attendees included such luminaries as Meyer Lansky, Ralph Capone, Charlie Fischetti and Frank Sinatra (U.S. Narcotics Bureau Report, undated). U.S. gangsters were not alone in these negotiations, but were actively assisted at every turn by high-ranking representatives of the Grau government.

Cuban congressmen Indalecio Pertierra (described in one FBI report as "Lucky Luciano's personal representative in Cuba") sponsored Luciano's immigration visa in 1946. Luciano stayed at the luxurious Miramar residence of Grau's army chief General Genevive Perez Damera, and was known to socialize frequently with Cuban congressmen Eduardo Suarez Rivas, Antonio and Francisco Prio (brothers of Grau's protégé, future President Carlos Prio) and other high ranking politicians. Senator Suarez Rivas had previously traveled from Havana to New York to attend Luciano's going away party.

The Grau regime went to great efforts to facilitate expansion of organized crime and smuggling on the island. In 1945 the government established a special new airline (Q Airlines, named for Grau crony Colonel Manuel Quevado) to move tourists and contraband between Havana and the United States. Quevado and army chief Perez Damera arranged for Q Airlines flights to go directly from Key West to Camp Colombia, a military installation outside of Havana, where immigration and customs inspections were waived. From there the tourists were transported to Havana's luxury hotels and casinos. In other words, Q Airlines essentially was given an official government license to smuggle on behalf Grau and the Auténtico Party. In a 1947 report, the U.S. Narcotics Bureau stated, "General Genevive Perez Damera made landing areas available in Cuba which were protected from government supervision and the airplanes were to be used for smuggling purposes." In addition to Quevado, a number of other high ranking Cuban congressmen were described as "concerned with this project with Luciano" (Ray Olivera, memo to Anslinger, March 26, 1947). By the end of the 1940s, Q Airlines had inaugurated daily flights from a number of Florida cities, and U.S. Narcotics Commissioner Anslinger told the *New York Times* that seizures of cocaine and heroin were occurring "on a scale unknown since before World War II" (*New York Times*, March 1949). By all accounts, these trends continued unabated following the return of Batista in the early 1950s.

Political Corruption

Corruption in the Auténtico regimes was not limited to facilitating the expansion of North American criminal syndicates and narcotics smuggling. Grau (and his successor Carlos Prio Socarras) also controlled extensive gambling revenues. Luciano and Frank Costello allegedly paid Congressman Indalecio Pertierra $50,000 for permission to operate a casino in the Hotel Presidente, with an undetermined percentage of the proceeds of the casino sent to Grau and his mistress Paulina (Report from Olivera to Anslinger, March 1947). Meyer Lansky and his subordinates continued to operate the casinos at the Jockey Club and the Montmartre Club together with Cuban officials such as Congressman Indalecio Pertierra. Exact figures earned by these joint investments in vice between Cuban politicians and North American gangsters are not available for this time period, but presumably many millions of dollars were involved.

These increasing riches from the vice trade also did not diminish Cuban politicians' efforts to plunder the national treasury. The Ministry of Education during the Auténtico era was known as a notorious source of graft and patronage, much of it allegedly directed to the armed gangs who controlled the campus of the University of Havana (Suchlicki, 1969). According to one FBI memo, this relationship became quite apparent when the Cuban government attempted to eliminate a number of sinecures from the Ministry in 1946,

> . . . [R]eliable sources in Havana, Cuba have reported that the Cuban Ministry of Education, since the beginning of the Grau regime, has been the source of thousands of political jobs. At one time there were reportedly 9,000 "botelleros" or holders of sinecures attached to this Ministry. For some months, the Ministry of Education has been paying out salaries far in excess of its financial appropriation and the Government realized that this

situation could not continue. Accordingly, some 4,000 employees were forced to resign during April, 1946, and 1500 more were to be cut off the payroll in May to enable the Ministry to operate within its budget. . . . As soon as the results of the conference [to eliminate jobs] were known, various revolutionary groups prepared to seize the Ministry of Education. At approximately 5 A.M. on May 10 a group of about thirty-five revolutionary organization members, armed with machine guns and small arms, took over the Ministry without resistance from the Police who were assigned to guard the building. The revolutionaries held the building until approximately 11 A.M. that morning, at which time they were assured by President Grau that none of them would lose their jobs (J. Edgar Hoover, Memo to Frederick B. Lyon June 4, 1946).

Officials from the Grau government also looted several workers' pension funds controlled by the government. According to Thomas (1998:746),"Despite its immense revenue the [Grau] government nevertheless embarked on the most daring and contemptible of its frauds— the theft of the reserve of non-governmental pension and social security funds lodged with the Treasury." According to a U.S. Embassy report from Havana in 1949 Grau did not deny that $175 million Cuban pesos had disappeared during his presidency, but claimed that the money was used to win the elections for his chosen successor, Carlos Prio. The Embassy report concluded on a relatively optimistic note, "The Cuban people, however, don't pay too much attention to these matters; they just take it for granted that the politicians in power must get rich quick one way or the other" (U.S. Embassy Report from Havana, January 1949). In March of 1951 Grau was formally indicted for misappropriation of over $40 million during his presidency (*New York Times* March nineteenth), though others estimate Grau may have stolen as much as $80 million (Bethel, 1969). The close relationship between Grau and organized crime groups in Havana was revealed when four masked gunmen broke into the prosecutor's office and stole all of the papers relating to Grau's indictment for misappropriation of funds. With the key evidence missing, the case was dismissed and Grau was never prosecuted.

The Prio Regime, 1948–1952

In November 1948 Grau's protégé, Carlos Prio Socarras (also of the Auténtico Party) was elected President of Cuba. Prio had previously served as Prime Minister under Grau, and was well-liked by United States officials for his anti-communist activities. In 1946 the Soviet Union shifted from its wartime alliance with the United States to an aggressively anti-American stance. At that time the Cuban communist party still maintained a formal alliance with the Prio's Auténtico Party, and the United States began to pressure Grau and Prio to distance themselves from their communist party supporters.

In May of 1947 Grau declared the Party illegal, and the Auténtico leadership began a ruthless purge of the Cuban Confederation of Labor. On July 29, Prio took over the labor confederation by force from Party leader Lazaro Peña and handed control to Auténtico Party trade unionists. Some reports allege that hired gunmen from radical student action groups (the ARG, the UIR, the MSR and other remnants of Antonio Guiteras' organization) were used by Grau and Prio to engineer this transfer of power. Ironically many of these groups had originally begun as radical leftist student groups affiliated with the Communist Party, but had since deteriorated into warring gangs devoted primarily to violence, extortion and blackmail (Suchlicki, 1969). In October, the Communist Party formally broke with the Auténticos, claiming they were "cruelly persecuted" by their former allies (Thomas, 1998).

Despite receiving several international honors, Prio's government remained as corrupt as his predecessors. One historian has estimated that Prio may have stolen as much as $90 million of public funds during his presidency (Paterson, 1994). Prio also invested heavily in Miami real estate developments with U.S. organized crime leader Santos Trafficante. These activities earned Prio fierce criticism from one of Cuba's most impassioned political reformers, Eddie Chibas[11] In June 1949, Chibas published an open letter to Prio stating,

> Tell me, Carlos Prio, how you can buy so many farms and build in them so many and various things while at the same time you say that there is no money and no material to build roads or carry out state public works, that there is nothing with which to pay the veterans of the War of Independence nor for the costs of the schools . . . tell me why you suddenly put at liberty the famous international drug trafficker whom you arrested in the Hotel Nacional with a cargo of drugs for the head of the secret police? (quoted in Thomas, 1998:762).

Prio and his followers were undeterred by these criticisms. Despite the fact that gambling was still illegal in Cuba, Prio and his brothers (one of whom was Minister of the Treasury) financed the reopening of the Sans Souci casino in a joint venture with several U.S. mobsters in the winter of 1950.

Health Trends under the Auténticos

As might be expected given the breadth and scope of political corruption in Cuba during the Auténtico years, Havana's public health infrastructure received little in the way of capital improvements. In addition to graft and sinecures in public works projects, corruption was endemic within the Ministry of Health. In the early fall of 1947 Grau's Minister of Health was assassinated by political gangsters (Thomas, 1998:755). The exact reasons for this killing are not specified by Thomas, but given the long-standing practice of diverting narcotics drugs from Ministry of Health stocks to North American organized crime groups it stands to reason that the killing was motivated by some dispute involving the drug trade.

Other reports from this time detail considerable neglect of basic health measures in Cuba's major cities during the Grau and Prio regimes. According to Phillips,

> Grau's public works program had failed to materialize; only a few streets in Havana had been paved; many projects were started but none ever seemed to be finished. Towns in the interior began to stage mass protest meetings against the waste of money and failure of the government to carry out announced projects ... graft was rampant in governmental departments, black markets flourished, and the public works program had broken down (1959:238).

Over twenty years earlier, during the Macahdo administration, the United State Public Health Service office in Havana had stated, "The scarcity of water has lasted twelve years and is getting worse. It is time something should be done." Despite the inauguration of three successive "revolutionary" regimes since that time, Havana's water supply remained contaminated. In 1947, the mayor valiantly tried to organize the construction of a new waterworks for the city, but was "blocked at every turn by politicians bent on collecting graft and the negligence of President Grau in providing money from the national treasury" (Phillips, 1959:240). Overwhelmed with anger and frustration at this political corruption and inertia, the mayor eventually committed suicide. By the time Carlos Prio took power in 1948, Cuba's urban infrastructure appeared to have declined even further. A report issued by the International Bank for Reconstruction and Development following a 1950 tour of Cuba also noted that while the private health sector in Cuba appeared adequate, the public health sector continued to suffer from neglect and mismanagement,

> From talks with Cubans, the impression was formed that Cuba has some of the best physicians and surgeons in the world, some admirable cooperative health schemes and some excellent hospitals. But the mission was often told that the administration of public health measures and of public hospitals leaves much to be desired . . . Traveling through the island, members of the commission could not fail to notice deficiencies in—and often complete lack of—municipal services, such as water supplies, sewers and paved streets. In many towns and communities the situation has become urgent and calls for serious measures. In some places, of course, much as been done by the government to improve these services. But because of a lack of any over-all programs, because of political favoritism, and of inept municipal governments, only a few communities at present enjoy a relatively adequate standard of municipal services (International Bank for Reconstruction and Development, 1950:449).

This report also described rather grim health conditions for the poor in Cuba in 1950. The authors claimed, for instance, that between eighty and ninety percent of the children in rural areas were infected with intestinal parasites—a situation that would have greatly facilitated malnutrition and infection in children. The same report also concluded that between 30–50 percent of the urban populations in Cuba (including in Havana) suffered from some form of malnutrition or vitamin deficiency. In rural areas, the commission estimated the percentage to be as high as 60 percent (International Bank for Reconstruction and Development Report on Cuba, 1950. Washington, DC p. 442).

These statistics raise some troubling questions. If a national government becomes so corrupt that its primary concerns are graft, embezzlement and facilitating the expansion of international organized crime rather than providing basic public health services to its population, do neighboring countries have an obligation to intervene on humanitarian grounds? The purposes of raising this question is to point out the tremendous difficulties Cuba's *caudillo* governments have posed for United States policy makers throughout the twentieth century. During the Platt era, repeated U.S. interventions (whether on humanitarian, imperialistic, or some combination of both) seemed only to increase Cuba's instability, violence, and anti-Americanism.

Nonintervention, on the other hand, hardly seemed a better alternative. U.S. inaction in the face of Cuba's social and political ills seemed to imply tacit American support for the destructive cycles of dictatorship, health decline and entrenched political corruption that emerged in Cuba following the abrogation of the Platt Amendment. Ironically, U.S. nonintervention in Cuban politics also bred intense anti-Americanism since it was viewed as covert support for corrupt dictatorships.

The Second Batista Regime, 1952–1959

On March 10, 1952 Fulgencio Batista staged a coup d'etat and ousted Carlos Prio Socarras from power. Realizing the army backed the coup, Prio quickly surrendered and fled to Mexico with several of his key advisors. Batista immediately made a clean sweep of all department chiefs in the police and army known to be loyal to Prio, instituted a powerful crackdown on the communist party, and raised salaries for the army in preparation for an extended military dictatorship (*New York Times*, March 10–13, 1952). He also dissolved the Cuban Confederation of Labor, and placed its (Auténtico) leaders under house arrest. Batista deported thirteen North American organized crime figures for illegal gambling activities and boasted of having broken an up a major narcotics smuggling ring allegedly bringing cocaine into Cuba (for the Auténtico leadership) via diplomatic pouch.[12]

The Gangster-State, Part 3

With the rival Auténticos effectively disenfranchised, Batista immediately began conferring with Meyer Lansky to expand organized crime activities on the island yet again. All forms of vice flourished in Havana at this time. Prostitution, pornography, narcotics, gambling (both legal and illegal) and gangland slayings were all common features of the city's landscape. As one *New York Times* report by Herbert Matthews noted in 1956,

... [T]here is no question that Cuba has the dubious distinction of being the most violent of all the Latin American nations. Nowhere in the hemisphere is life so cheap. ... Those in power are able to enrich themselves and hence the temptations to fight for political power are great. These days, for instance, there are four illegal lotteries in Havana with two drawings a day. It is estimated that the profits from these lotteries come to about $1 million daily. This in addition to the legal lotteries part of whose proceeds go to many men connected with the Government, including the Army. There is a public works program under way amounting to about $350 million and in Cuba it is notorious that not all the money that is budgeted goes into the public works. Consequently much of the violence in Cuba is simply an effort by the outs to get in and thus to share the spoils of office. However, there is a genuine revolutionary and often patriotic element in the violence as well as sordid gangsterism (November 4, 1956).

Batista soon acted to expand these activities even further by legalizing gambling and passing laws subsidizing hotel construction in the tourism industry. Between 1952 and 1959 over ten new luxury hotel casinos opened in Cuba, all operated by North American organized crime figures who paid vast sums to Batista's henchmen to obtain gambling concessions. Batista's favored military officers were strongly encouraged to participate in these activities. One of Batista's army commanders (allegedly a close associate of the General) authorized seventeen new casinos to open on his very first night as head of the provincial military post in Santa Clara in 1959 (FBI Memo on Cuban Revolutionary Activities, February 5, 1959).

Batista and his henchmen made millions in payoffs from these arrangements. In order to obtain a gambling license, tourism officials required an "unofficial" $25,000 payoff, plus another official $25,000 "donation" to the tourist commission. In some cases older hotel casinos were assessed an unofficial $100,000 fee after they completed renovations. Government officials were also given about $3000 a month per casino in "protection" money. The bolita, an unofficial lottery, brought in another $175,000 to $300,000 per week for the government, which (according to one FBI informant) was divided equally between the Chief of Police, the head of the Detective Bureau on the police force, and Batista's wife. The Cuban government also received between 30 and 50 percent of all slot machine revenues in Cuba. During the tourist season, the machines at the Hotel Nacional *alone* brought in between five and six thousand dollars per week. One FBI report estimated that the chief of police in Havana alone earned approximately \$3–4 million per year in illegal payoffs.[13] Carlos Alberto Montaner has described Batista's second regime as a wholesale keptocracy that surpassed all previous levels of corruption in Cuba,

[Batista] stole, permitted stealing, and benefited from others' stealing, with a neurotic frenzy. Ten percent of the budget from the Department of Public Works ended up in his pockets. . . . With his close relatives he shared the gambling profits (legal and illegal). He would sell sinecures, decrees, favors, customhouse directorships, government positions, and any other 'merchandise' within the reach of an uncontrollable and dishonest ruler. It must be acknowledged that he did not invent such practices, and that his predecessors did the same things, but Batista carried corruption to unheard-of limits (1981:6).

Health Trends under Batista, 1952–1959

Batista's return to power in Cuba was heralded with traditional health propaganda. In a pamphlet published a year after his coup, Batista claimed that one of his goals in forcibly seizing control of the Cuban state was to rescue Cuban health from the hands of the corrupt Auténticos and restore it to the standards that prevailed during the so-called "golden era of sanitation" (Ministerio de Salubridad y Asistencia Social, 1953). Batista's secretary of sanitation echoed these sentiments, detailing how the coup was motivated by Batista's deeply-felt patriotic desire to personally resolve Cuba's health problems:

Major General Fulgencio Batista y Zaldivar, Honorable President of the Republic of Cuba and Commander in Chief of the Revolutions of September 4 [1933] and March 10 [1952] has a very personal preoccupation with the health of his people. . . . His vast program or plan in this area is not something that is readily achieved in just one year. He hopes and desires to achieve what Carlos Finlay, Juan Guiteras, Enrique Barnet and López de Valle dreamed [for Cuban health care]. A project this grand requires a sustained and continuous effort, for a time longer than the twelve months that we have been able to act (Ministerio de Salubridad y Asistencia Social, 1953).

Were Batista's health programs effective? Or was this simply more propaganda intended to divert attention away from Batista's dictatorial government, corruption and cozy relationship with North American gangsters? There are few alternative sources of information available for this time period, but one *New York Times* article from June of 1952 did note that popular discontent against Batista was rising due to the lack of progress in sanitation and infrastructure improvements,

> . . . [T]he people are becoming impatient over the slowness of the Government in solving many problems which have been accumulating over the past years such as in Havana, an acute water shortage, a lack of a drainage system in the suburbs, a shortage of meat, a lack of efficient sanitation measures and the failure to start necessary public works throughout the island (June 27, 1952).

Unfortunately, there was little attempt on the part of the U.S. media to thoroughly investigate these allegations. The *New York Times* devoted nearly all of its Cuban coverage in the 1950s to either the tourism industry or the anti-Batista rebellions organized by deposed President Carlos Prio Socarras (and later Fidel Castro). Batista's Ministry of Health did release data on health trends, but these figures must be viewed with some suspicion given the long-standing tradition in Cuba of distorting health data to justify dictatorial government. Interestingly enough, some of the most credible descriptions of health trends in the late 1950s come from early documents published by Fidel Castro's own Ministry of Health, released shortly after the 1959 revolution.

Notes

1. Exact dollar amounts of these payoffs are not available for this time period. By the 1950s, however, the FBI was collecting information regarding financial relationships between North American gangsters and Cuban politicians. These figures will be presented later in this chapter.
2. One of Beals' most famous works *The Crime of Cuba*, written in the early 1930s to protest Machado's dictatorial government, as well as his collusion with North American capitalists.
3. Grau would later be elected President from 1944-1948.
4. A perhaps unintended consequence of this legislation was to make the University a haven for criminals and smugglers. Gunfights and assassinations were common on campus throughout the 1940s.
5. Guiteras was not the only revolutionary killed at this time. Killed with him were Venezuelan General Carlos Aponte (a former aide to Sandino in Nicaragua) and José Mas. They were allegedly attempting to flee Cuba in a yacht belonging to

deposed *caudillo* Mario Menocal. After his death, Guiteras' North American mother, Maria Theresa Holmes, described him as "a great revolutionary against the forces of capitalism and yankee imperialism" (*New York Times* May 9, 1935).

6. Batista was the unofficial ruler of Cuba from 1934-1940, and was formally elected president from 1940-1944. In the 1944 elections he was voted out of power in favor of Grau san Martín and the Auténtico Party. Grau ruled until 1948, when his chosen successor Carlos Prio Socarras was elected. Prio was deposed by Batista in a coup in 1952.

7. In 1935 the *New York Times* noted the existence of seventeen rival student-led left wing parties in Cuba. These included the formal Communist Party, the ABC Radical (a violent leftist group organized out of the ABC); the Student Directorate; the left wing of the Student Directorate; the Young Pioneers League (run by the Communist Party); the Anti-Imperialist League; several nationalistic groups called "50, 75, and 80 percent organizations" devoted to nationalism in labor practices; the Student Left Organization; student gangster groups known only as TNT and X (allegedly led by Carlos Hevia); the Cuban Medical Federation (led by a branch of the communist party); the Cuban Revolutionary Party (led by Grau San Martín); the Grupo Antorcha; and the Young Communist League (*New York Times,* March 1935).

8. Fidel Castro was an early member of the UIR and was described by many people who knew him at that time as a "political gangster" (see Thomas, 1998; Geyer, 1984).

9. It should be emphasized that these reports were not official health propaganda released by the government, but private reports from local health officials to the national Ministry in Havana. They are located in the provincial archives in Santiago-de-Cuba and in the Carlos Finlay Library in Havana.

10. Guillermo Cabrera-Infante has stated of Grau, "He seized the confused ideas of Guiteras and made them even more confused" (1994:139).

11. Chibas had previously criticized Carlos Prio for the close relationship his brother Paco maintained with U.S. mafia chief Lucky Luciano. During Luciano's visit in Havana, Prio and Chibas fought a duel over these accusations. Both were slightly wounded.

12. Batista's reorganization of gambling is detailed in various FBI files from Havana in the late 1950s, the drug smuggling ring is described in an article in *Focus* Magazine (volume 2, number 8) August, 1952. Batista's crackdown on the communist party and labor groups is described in various *New York Times* articles from 1952.

13. All of these figures are taken from various FBI reports from Cuba between 1952-1959.

10

Revolutionaries in Power, 1959–

Prior to 1959, all Cuban revolutions were inaugurated with great fanfare, but in the end resulted in little more than a continuation of the militarization, *caudillismo* and corruption of previous regimes. The revolutionaries of 1906 were primarily concerned with plundering the national treasury. The revolutionaries of 1917 were much the same. Even the chaotic, impassioned revolution against Machado in the early 1930s led only to deepening cycles of graft, corruption and political-gangster violence in the 1940s and 1950s. By the time Batista returned to power in his 1952 "revolution," the term appeared to signify little more than an armed takeover of the public sector, including its gambling and smuggling rackets. Did the Castro revolutionaries reiterate this pattern? Or did 1959, unlike earlier Cuban revolutions, represent a truly radical break from the past? As long as political dissent in Cuba remains so heavily criminalized, and independent investigation of the Castro regime's programs continues to be prohibited, a full accounting of the 1959 Revolution's place in history cannot be made. Nonetheless, a casual appraisal does reveal a number of important continuities as well as some key divergences (especially with respect to health and disease) between the Castro revolutionaries and their predecessors.

Caudillismo, Militarization and Health (1959–1989)

Like earlier *caudillo* regimes, the Castro revolutionaries have dramatically increased the size and scope of the military in Cuba[1], and have used the army to establish control of the country's economic production. By the late 1960s, every enterprise of the country was effectively nationalized by the revolutionary leadership, and the Cuban military grew to be the largest per population in the Western hemisphere (Fernández, 1989). Numerous paramilitary organizations, such as the Committees for the Defense of the Revolution and various youth organizations, further supplemented the regular armed forces.

The Castro revolutionaries have also reiterated earlier patterns of rule in their complete intolerance of political dissent, bitter conflicts with exiled political coalitions in Miami, and international arms and narcotics trafficking.[2] Furthermore, there has been a consistent practice by the regime of using positive health data to win international support and divert attention from the violence and authoritarianism of *caudillo* rule. In this sense, the criticisms voiced by one journalist in the 1920s against the Machado dictatorship still appear quite relevant today,

> Thus the answer to the charge that General Machado's friends had abused the Constitution to continue him in office for another six years was to point to a gleaming new hospital; the answer to the charge that opponents of the government had been denied opportunity to organize a party was an immaculate new high school; the answer to the charge that the President has burdened the country with heavy taxation to carry out his ambitious program was a model industrial city where the workers live in better homes than they enjoy in the United States (*New York Times*, October 21, 1930).

Unlike the Machado regime, however, some of the health initiatives of the Castro revolutionaries have been quite substantial. The changes in clinical medicine engineered by the revolutionary government have received the most sustained attention (and praise) in international public health and medical anthropology literature, but the most significant transformation in the health sector since 1959 has probably been the aggressive militarization of public health. As previously mentioned, the ability of clinical practitioners to prevent epidemics of infectious disease is often quite limited. Activities such as vaccination, water purification, sewage disposal, insect and rodent control, housing and nutrition are beyond the domain of clinical medicine. Instead, these disease prevention measures are typically organized and executed within the domain of government public health and welfare programs.

Before 1959, Cuba's public health sector was deeply dysfunctional due to long-standing patterns of political corruption, violence and instability. While private sector medicine on the island was quite good (though poorly distributed), individual doctors were powerless to undertake the massive engineering and public works programs necessary to control pathogenic microbes and prevent disease outbreaks. Advances in medical technology in the mid twentieth century such as vaccines and antibiotics were greatly useful in controlling infectious diseases on the island, but offered little as far as prevention.

One of the first acts of the Castro revolutionaries was to place the rebel army in charge of public health and public works in Cuba's major cities. A number of important sanitation improvements were also undertaken by the army during this time: waterworks were renovated, sewers built, streets paved and a house-to-house health census and mosquito eradication campaign (similar to the ones conducted during the American occupation in 1898) were implemented (see Danielson, 1981). In 1959 approximately $12,000 was spent per month to hire a brigade of inspectors to eradicate mosquitos in urban areas. In 1960s, this was increased to a force involving seventy brigades with over 400 inspectors (MINISAP, 1960).

By the mid-1960s, paramilitary neighborhood organizations such as the CDR (Committees for the Defense of the Revolution) were increasingly tasked with community health outreach and epidemiological surveillance activities (see CDR, 1964; 1966). In addition to patrolling neighborhoods for signs of political subversion or dissent, the CDR were also expected to keep track of pregnant women, to engage in health education regarding the importance of prenatal care, provide advice on breast feeding and to register births once they occurred. The CDR also engaged in other types of health outreach including vaccination, nutrition, general household hygiene, mosquito control, and water purification (CDR, 1966). In rural areas, where formal CDR organization was impractical because of low population density, other mass organizations such as the ANAP (the association of peasant farmers) or the FMC (the Federation of Cuban Women) took over these and other public health efforts (MINISAP, 1974; MINISAP, 1986). Great emphasis was also placed on constructing new hospitals and health facilities. By 1963, 122 rural health centers and forty-two new rural hospitals had been established (Danielson, 1981:133).

These developments undoubtedly resulted in significant health improvements in Cuba in the 1960s and 1970s. In previous generations, resources allocated for health programs had been diverted into the pockets of corrupt national and local officials. The substitution of an authoritarian, militarized public health sector with an emphasis on civic honesty meant that resources allocated for health improvements actually reached their target populations (see Danielson, 1977; 1979; 1981; Guttmacher and Danielson, 1979; Padula, 1993; Thomas, 1998). As Hugh Thomas stated in the early 1970s, "Everywhere [in Cuba] there has been a marked increase in hygiene and sanitation" (1971:1426).

Health Transitions (1959–1989)

Unfortunately, it is difficult to ascertain exactly how much health in Cuba improved after 1959. Cuban exile coalitions and the Castro government have both reiterated earlier generations of *caudillo* wars by using health propaganda to attack and discredit one another. In the early 1960s, a Cuban Medical Association in Exile was formed in Miami that released a number of publications with such provocative titles as "The Great Tragedy of Health in Cuba," and "The Terrible Crisis of Medicine in Castro's Cuba" (Castellanos, 1962a; Castellanos, 1962b). In 1964 the Cuban Student Directorate (in exile) also issued a report claiming that hepatitis, syphilis, smallpox, malnutrition and starvation had all increased dramatically in Cuba due to the importation of shoddy medical equipment and poorly trained (and unclean) personnel from the Soviet Union and China,

> In 1957–1958 congenital syphilis was almost extinguished [in Cuba] due to the ample use of penicillin and the anti-venereal disease campaign. Since Castro took over, the percentage of syphilis has continually increased and all Children's Hospitals have tremendous amounts of cases as in 1930. The immorality and the foreign population coming from countries of low sanitary conditions like China, Algeria, Korea, Egypt, Russia . . . etc. and the lack of penicillin explains the increase in the number of congenital syphilis [cases] (DRE, 1964).

Fulgencio Batista also produced his own critiques of Castro's health programs from exile, in such books as *The Growth and Decline of the Cuban Republic* (1964) and *Cuba Betrayed* (1961). In these works, Batista proudly iterates his accomplishments as President of Cuba, and accuses the Castro regime of destroying health on the island.

In Cuba, a number of MINISAP publications were produced to

respond to these attacks, describing tremendous health progress by the revolutionary government. The first of these was released in 1960, and sharply criticized Batista's health programs for worsening Cuba's "misery, hunger, and oppression" at the hands of U.S. imperialists. The pamphlet concluded by stating, "In nineteen months of revolution, Cuba has advanced more in the area of sanitation than in all the rest of its fifty eight years as a republic" (MINISAP, 1960). An elaborate recitation of statistics (highly reminiscent of Batista's description of his health programs above) was then provided, enumerating the number of sanitary brigades formed by the new regime, along with statistical overviews of anti-mosquito programs and investment in hospitals and health facilities.

In 1968 and 1969 MINISAP released new publications to announce a "revolutionary offensive" in health, and to chart the revolution's progress in areas of health and sanitation. Each of these documents detailed the misery and disease Cuba had endured under "imperialism" and described the efforts of the revolutionary regime to improve conditions. Additional pamphlets were published by MINISAP in 1974 and 1988. All of these MINISAP documents used health statistics to portray the dramatic health improvements that ostensibly took place after the 1959 Revolution. Curiously enough, however, the statistical portrayal of the "pre-revolutionary era" is quite different in each of these MINISAP documents, as well as in more recent articles (based on current MINISAP statistics) that have appeared in U.S. medical journals. Reviewing these documents in sequence offers some insight into the actual changes in health conditions that have taken place since the late 1950s.

In early MINISAP documents, health conditions in the late 1950s are typically portrayed much more favorably than they are in contemporary publications—a pattern that suggests the revolutionary regime has strategically reinvented certain aspects of the pre-revolutionary past to exaggerate its own contributions to Cuba's favorable health profile. This trend becomes apparent when these publications are examined in sequence. In 1963, only four years after the Castro brothers took power, the Cuban Ministry of Health released a pamphlet comparing Cuba's infant mortality and death rates from gastritis and enteritis (leading causes of infant mortality in the Third World) with those of other Latin American countries. According to these figures, Cuba's infant mortality rate was actually quite low during the Batista era compared with other Latin American countries, ranging between thirty-seven and fifty per 1,000 live births (depending on which source is consulted—the figure of thirty-seven per 1,000 comes from the original MINISAP documents, as well as the Statistical Abstract of the United States for 1957, the figure of fifty comes from more recent MINISAP documents). According to Schneider et al. (2002) both of these figures are substantially lower than the average infant mortality rate in Latin American at this time, which was over ninety per 1,000 live births.[3] The infant mortality rate for Cuba in 1959 was also substantially lower than the rates that prevail in many third world countries today. In 2002 Pakistan's infant mortality rate was estimated to be between 78–80 per 1,000 live births, and Ethiopia's was well over 100 per 1000 live births (http://www.indexmundi.com).

The 1963 MINISAP pamphlet also described three of Cuba's five leading causes of death in 1959 (*before* the revolution) as heart disease, cancer and stroke—in other words, a high proportion of the island's mortality at this time appeared to be from chronic rather than infectious disease. This implies that Cuba in these years had already undergone some degree of demographic modernization, or a shift in mortality patterns from infectious to chronic disease, consistent with Batista's claim that health conditions during his reign were not overwhelmingly bad, and outbreaks of infectious disease were adequately controlled.

These early statistics released by MINISAP do not suggest that Cuba's health profile before 1959 was typical of extreme underdevelopment, as the Castro regime implies today. Furthermore, the fact that the figures cited by MINISAP for the pre-revolutionary era themselves have changed substantially over the past forty years implies that the present government is deliberately attempting to erase evidence of Cuba's health gains in the 1940s and 1950s and take exclusive credit for Cuba's twentieth century demographic modernization. The follow tables offer a comparison of health data from MINISAP from the early 1960s through the 1990s.

There are several ways to interpret these statistical discrepancies. First of all, it is conceivable that *all* of these figures are correct, in which case it would appear that diphtheria was not a major public health problem in Cuba until 1960, when a major epidemic (which would have been the largest in Cuban history) must have taken place. Given that there are no news reports of a major outbreak of diphtheria

TABLE 10.1
Reinventing the "Pre-Revolutionary" Past: Diphtheria

Source	Year in Question	Cases Reported
MINISAP, 1963	1962	20
MINISAP, 1963	1963	10
Gilpin [MINISAP], 1991	1960	300–500
MINISAP, 1997[4]	"pre-revolutionary era"	600 (*for Santiago only*)
Diphtheria Statistics from Earlier Regimes:		
Ortega, 1940	1925 (*for Santiago only*)	3
Batista, 1964	1958	85

at this time (there were still American journalists reporting from Havana in 1960), this scenario seems unlikely.

An alternative explanation would be that the statistics from earlier regimes (i.e., the Ortega and Batista reports) were incorrect, and that the rates reported by MINISAP in 1991 for 1960 (i.e., the 300–500 cases per year) represent the true extent of the pre-revolutionary incidence of diphtheria, which the revolution subsequently (and dramatically) combated, thus reducing the rates to the minimal twenty cases per year reported for 1962.

This scenario also seems unlikely in that the years between 1959 and 1962 were years of intense social and economic upheaval and the newly empowered revolutionary government had not yet had time to effectively consolidate its power, much less initiate the kind of nation wide public health campaign necessary to reduce diphtheria rates from 300–500 cases per year down to only twenty. Also, between 1959 and 1962 there was a tremendous exodus of doctors and other trained health workers (some estimates claim as high as 50 percent) from Cuba, meaning that any public health efforts would have been severely constrained by personnel shortages. According to a speech given by Fidel Castro in the summer of 2005, Cuba was severely short of health care workers in the early 1960s, and "only a handful of students graduated as doctors during the first years following the triumph of the Revolution" (Castro Ruz, 2005). In this speech, Castro notes that it took until almost 1970 for the number of new doctors trained to roughly equal those who left in the early years of the revolution, meaning that the entire decade of the 1960s would have seen severe shortages of medical personnel. Ross Danielson has also stated that it was not until

1961 that the revolutionary government developed its own plan for a "comprehensive national system of health services (1979:143)." Furthermore, this plan was not fully implemented for several years, and then underwent still more substantial revisions in 1965 to make it more in keeping with the Czech and East European model of health services endorsed by the Soviet advisors working in Cuba at this time.

The third way of interpreting these figures would be to conclude that the Castro regime has strategically reinvented the health of the pre-revolutionary era (essentially creating a past epidemic of diphtheria) to be more in keeping with the rhetoric of the revolutionary leadership and the predictions of dependency theory with respect to health. The original 1963 MINISAP document, for instance, appears to have been designed to show the revolution's impressive health achievements in its first four years of rule (i.e., reducing diphtheria incidence by half—from twenty cases per year down to ten). In other words, this early document appears very much in keeping with the long standing tradition of generating health propaganda to justify an armed seizure of power. These original figures for diphtheria, however, (i.e., only ten cases in the entire country) left little room for health progress in this area following the transition to communism, making it necessary to retroactively add diphtheria cases to the "pre-revolutionary" era so that greater progress in combating this infection could be demonstrated.

According to the original 1969 MINISAP statistics, polio rates actually appeared to increase dramatically following the revolution, then declined sharply in 1962–1963 after a comprehensive vaccination program was put into place. This initial increase, however, is not mentioned in contemporary texts, which inevitably describe the immediate eradication of polio by the revolutionary government (Gilpin, 1991; Waitzkin, 1983). Furthermore, contemporary MINISAP accounts appear to use the highest ever incidence of polio recorded in Cuba as if it represented an average for the entire 1900–1959 time period. In reality it appears more likely that polio rates were quite variable from year to year. Batista, for instance, claimed to have initiated a widespread vaccination campaign that dramatically reduced polio rates from 265 cases down to fifty-six cases between 1955 and 1956 (Batista, 1964). Again, it is difficult to ascertain whether this was a legitimate public health campaign or another manifestation of the ongoing tendency to justify an armed seizure of power by generative favorable health statistics.

TABLE 10.2
Polio

Source	Year in Question	Cases Reported
MINISAP, 1969	1958	104
MINISAP, 1969	1959	288
MINISAP, 1969	1961	342
MINISAP, 1969	1962	46
Gilpin, 1991 [MINISAP]	"pre-revolutionary"	300–500 per year
MINISAP, 1997	"pre-revolutionary" (*for Santiago only*)	300 per year

Polio Statistics from Earlier Regimes:

Source	Year in Question	Cases Reported
Mencia, 1936	1934	434
Mencia, 1936	1935	179
Mencia, 1936	1936	60
Batista, 1964	1955	265
Batista, 1964	1956	56

In March of 1961 a small article in the *New York Times* reported that the city of Guantanamo had been stricken with an outbreak of polio and three children had died. Vaccine supplies in the city were supposedly exhausted, and President Kennedy instructed medical personnel at the U.S. naval base at Guantanamo to rush a supply of polio vaccine by ambulance to the stricken city. The following day, Fidel Castro responded with an angry tirade in which he accused Kennedy of "imperialist objectives" in sending polio vaccine to Cuba, and insisted that no outbreak had occurred, "Denying that there had been a polio outbreak in Cuba or that Cuban officials had asked for help, the Ministry [of public health] said Mr. Kennedy's announcement was "filled with bad faith" (*New York Times*, March 10, 1961). This assertion is contradicted by MINISAP's own statistics, which clearly show evidence of a significant increase in polio cases in 1961.

In addition to the significant difference between MINISAP's 1968 reports of enteritis and gastritis and the figures given in 1991 and 1997, there is another major discrepancy with contemporary accounts. According to MINISAP's 1968 report, gastritis and enteritis were the third leading cause of death in Cuba in 1962, behind heart disease and cancer. Yet, according to Guttmacher and Danielson (1979:89), "Diarrheal diseases, including gastroenteritis, were *the leading causes of*

TABLE 10.3
Gastritis and Enteritis

Source	Year in Question	Deaths Reported
MINISAP, 1963	1959	2,887
MINISAP, 1968	1962	3,592
MINISAP, 1968	1963	2,727
MINISAP, 1968	1966	1,532
Gilpin, 1991 [MINISAP]	1962	4,147
MINISAP, 1997	"pre-revolutionary era" (*Santiago only*)	9,000

death in 1957" [emphasis added]. It seems unlikely that heart disease and cancer could have replaced gastritis and enteritis as leading causes of death in only five (very turbulent) years, before the revolutionary health care system had even been put into place. Furthermore, according to even earlier MINISAP statistics (1963), Cuba's rates of gastritis and enteritis were already some of the lowest in Latin America in 1957—two years *before* the revolution.

What these historical materials suggest is that Cuba appears to have been (in terms of health and sanitation) a healthier place in the Batista years than most contemporary representations of this period imply. This is not to suggest that there was *no* ill health or underdevelopment in Cuba prior to the revolution, only that there was quite likely very uneven development between rural and urban areas. This distinction, however, is important in understanding population health trends.

First of all, if health and sanitation conditions in urban areas were improving, it can be assumed that epidemics of infectious disease

TABLE 10.4
Mortality rates for Gastritis and Enteritis in Latin America, 1957–1960
[Source: MINISAP, 1963]

Country	Rate
Venezuela	62.2
Guatemala	233.2
Dominican Republic	202.6
Ecuador	136.3
Costa Rica	120.2
Nicaragua	100.3
Cuba	**43.3**

TABLE 10.5
Leading causes of death in Cuba, 1959
[Source: MINISAP, 1963]

Disease	# of Deaths	Rate/100,000 habitantes
1. Heart Disease	9,531	145.1
2. Cancer	5,810	87.2
3. Gastritis, enteritis	2,887	43.3
4. Cerebrovascular disease (i.e., stroke)	2,761	32.5
5. Influenza and Pneumonia	2,163	32.5

were relatively uncommon in Cuba in the 1950s. The reason for this is that epidemics of most infectious diseases occur in cities—rural areas simply do not have the population densities to sustain large-scale epidemics. Secondly, as many authors have pointed out, Cuba in the 1950s was already significantly urbanized—most people lived in cities and towns. One estimate, for instance, held that almost 80 percent of Cuba's population lived in urban areas as far back as 1936—a trend that was often said to date from the Spanish policy of *reconcentración* during the war of independence (Mencia, 1936).

Theodore Draper (1964), Nicholas Eberstadt (1986) and Sergio Diaz-Briquets (1986) have also argued that the Castro regime has deliberately sought to distort the extent of Cuba's underdevelopment in the 1950s in order to amplify its own contribution to the process of demographic modernization. Effective understanding of these dynamics, however, is greatly complicated by the fact that a number of anti-Castro activists have sought to distort the level of Cuba's development in the 1950s in order to effectively challenge the Castro regime's progressive rhetoric. Draper (1964:103) has criticized both of these practices as follows,

... [A] social interpretation of the Cuban revolution must begin with a view of a Cuban society that is far more urban, far less agrarian, far more middle class, far less backward, than it has been made to appear. ... In fact ... it would be far more helpful to think of Cuba as an unevenly developed country, with a backward hinterland that lagged further and further behind, and a middle class sector almost too large for the economy to sustain. In such a society, it is possible to manipulate statistics to emphasize extreme backwardness or extreme progressiveness, depending on which end of the scale is being manipulated. But the tendency to judge a country in terms of its least developed areas has even less to commend it than the tendency to judge it in terms of its most developed.

Revolutionary Medicine (1959–1989)

While the Castro regime's early militarization of the health sector has probably been the most significant factor in improving health since the late 1950s, the changes in clinical medicine also merit discussion. Both of these domains (public health and clinical medicine) underwent similar processes of militarization in the 1960s. Clinical practitioners have now become absorbed into the state public health infrastructure, and are viewed as "soldiers" who battle disease through clinical interventions and public health outreach.

The reorganization and militarization of clinical medicine began with the establishment of polyclinics in the mid-1960s. These centralized health centers were the focal point for medical practice in Cuba until the mid-1970s. At that time, a critical restructuring of health facilities was undertaken. The result was the creation of "medicine in the community." One of the key innovations of this system was a process called "sectorization" whereby the entire population was broken down into health sectors to be served by a physician-nurse team based out of the area polyclinic. Sectorization attempted to integrate clinical medicine and public health outreach by making the nurse-physician team responsible for the health of the entire community sector.

In the 1980s, the Medicine in the Community was expanded into the Family Doctor Program. This program was also intended to break down barriers between doctors and patients, by making physicians members of the communities they served. By living among their patients, the family doctor was supposedly better able to understand and address local health problems. Public health outreach was further integrated into clinical medicine with the adoption of the neighborhood health census into family medical practice. Family doctors in Cuba are expected to conduct a health census of their neighborhoods in order to keep track of local health trends and to better monitor patients with chronic conditions, such as diabetes or hypertension (see Feinsilver, 1993; Waitzkin and Britt, 1989; Guttmacher and Danielson, 1979). Family doctors often work together with paramilitary organizations such as the CDR to maintain local health and sanitation standards.

These changes in public health and clinical medicine, particularly the broadening of medical intervention to include issues of nutrition and housing, have been viewed as favorable by most international observers (see Feinsilver, 1993; Waitzkin and Britt, 1989; Nayeri, 1995; A. Chomsky, 2000). There are, however, also tremendous costs associated with militarizing public health and medicine in this way that have not been factored into these analyses. Medicine, for instance, is no longer an autonomous profession in Cuba. It is organized by the state into an intensely rigid, bureaucratic, hierarchical system. As a result, Cuban medicine has the potential to be intensely dehumanizing. Doctors and patients have no right to privacy in clinical interactions, and all health-related activities are subject to governmental intrusion to make sure they are in keeping with national health goals established by the Ministry of Public Health, and ideological goals established by the Communist Party or the revolutionary leadership.

The militarization of clinical medicine in Cuba means that there is no concept of patients' rights, and no tradition of informed consent[5] or right to refuse treatment. All of these rights form the cornerstone of medical ethics and clinical practice guidelines in most Western countries (see Jonsen, Siegler, Winslade, 2002). In Cuba, health goals, practice standards and medical directives are dictated by the Ministry of Health to individual clinicians, who must enforce them regardless of the preferences of individual patients. This has resulted in complete erosion of personal privacy and physician autonomy, as well as continued expansion of government power into such historically private realms as sexuality, reproduction and family dynamics.[6] This authoritarian approach is clearly visible in Cuba's repressive treatment of HIV patients, who have typically been incarcerated in sanitaria. Today, Cuba's AIDS sanitaria are described as "voluntary," yet during my time on the island, it was not uncommon to hear anecdotal reports of State Security officers removing HIV positive individuals from their homes by force (for various discussions of Cuba's HIV policy, see Hansen and Groce, 2003; Scheper-Hughes, 1993; Perez-Stable, 1991; Burr, 1997).

People who resist Cuba's health dictates (whether patients or practitioners) are at risk of being labeled "counterrevolutionaries" and punished accordingly. In the early 1960s, for instance, male homosexuality was viewed as incompatible with the revolution, and many gay men were incarcerated in rural internment camps where they were

subjected to medical-political "reeducation" that forced them to conform
to Hispanic heterosexual behavior norms. As Montaner has described,

> Camps of forced labor were instituted with all speed to "correct" such
> deviations [as homosexuality] . . . Verbal and physical mistreatment, shaved
> heads, work from dawn to dusk, hammocks, dirt floors, scarce food . . . The
> camps became increasingly crowded as the methods of arrest became more
> expedient. . . . The detainees were often young communists who were struck
> with the realization that the sexual expression and the ideology they had
> chosen were incompatible. Nobody was safe from sexual espionage
> (1981:144).

These practices have much in common with the mandatory "reha-
bilitation" or "reeducation" of political dissidents in Cuba, who continue to be incarcerated or forced into exile for challenging the regime's
dictates or for minor deviations from the Party line. Just as psychiatry
was co-opted into a force of control by the state in the former Soviet
Union, dissidents or other nonconformists in Cuba continue to be subjected to political-medical coercion (see Bloch and Reddaway, 1984;
Brown and Lago, 1991).

Even today, family doctors in Cuba are expected to keep records
describing the "political integration" of each family in their neighborhoods. Political integration refers to such activities as participation in
volunteer labor brigades, membership in mass organizations like the
FMC or CDR, as well as an exemplary work record. This survey
overlaps with other workplace and community programs of social and
political surveillance. The CDR, for instance, polices neighborhoods
for any potentially counterrevolutionary activities, while workplace
vigilance organizations monitor employees and mandate their participation in volunteer labor brigades, political rallies and parades. Epidemiological surveillance has thus become juxtaposed with political surveillance, and health professionals are expected to tend to the "health
of the revolution" by monitoring their communities for signs of political dissent and nonconformity as well as physical disease.

Cuban doctors still receive years of military training as part of their
medical education—training that emphasizes hierarchy, rank, and un-
questioning obedience to authorities. One introductory textbook, for
instance, (Rigol et al., 1994:28) described the role of the revolutionary
doctor as emblematic of "*un militante de la salud*" ("a health militant"). Another source revealed that the standard medical school cur-

riculum includes several semesters of mandatory classes in *"preparación militar"*—or military training (MINISAP, 1979). This training is designed to underscore the role of the physician in the war against imperialism and underdevelopment.

The family doctor is also supposed to comport himself or herself as an exceptionally ideal revolutionary—fervent, loyal, dedicated, and altruistic, and of course, completely intolerant of counterrevolutionaries or dissidents. One description of the ideal revolutionary doctor, for instance, included such personal traits as "simplicity, modesty, and honor" as well as "patriotic-military preparation necessary for the defense of the revolution and socialism on the national or international scale" (MINISAP, 1979:39). In terms of specific ideology, the physician is expected to embrace Marxist-Leninist theory and an appropriately "proletariat" attitude,

> In the formation of this [ideal revolutionary] doctor, with respect to political aspects, we must train him to confront the problems of the country: the defense of the fatherland, the call of internationalism, the development of a proletariat consciousness, the adoption of working class interests, so that he begins to have a clear conception of his role as a scientific worker, without elitist positions and with a just valorization of the workers who produce the material wealth . . . of society (MINISAP, 1979:56).

The authoritarian dimensions of Cuba's medical system even extend internationally as well. In 2000, two Cuban physicians sent abroad on a "medical mission" to Africa attempted to defect to the United States, and were kidnapped and forced onto an airplane by Cuban and Zimbabwean security personnel (DeYoung, 2000; Rodriguez and Martinez, 2000).

The Special Period (1989-)

The abrupt collapse of the Soviet Union in the early 1990s led to a dramatic economic crisis for Cuba. Between 1989 and 1993 the gross domestic product in Cuba contracted by almost 35 percent, leading to severe shortages of consumer goods and major fiscal deficits. According to Jorge Pérez-López, "merchandise exports contracted by 78.9 percent, and imports by 75.6 percent" between 1989 and 1993 (2002:509). These sharp economic declines imposed many hardships on Cuban families, and an epidemic of nutritional deficiency disease resulted from widespread food scarcity (see Feinsilver, 1993; Román, 1994).

To cope with this economic crisis, Fidel Castro inaugurated a "Special Period in Time of Peace" in the early 1990s. A range of new policies were introduced designed to liberalize the Cuban economy and encourage foreign investment. By 1997, a Cuban Chamber of Commerce guide listed over 200 new sociedad anonimas eager to attract foreign partners (Cuban Chamber of Commerce, 1997). Free farmers markets were reopened, and tourism was encouraged as a means for the regime to earn hard currency. Between 1990 and 2000, the number of foreigners tourists traveling to Cuba increased from an average of 340,000 per year to over 1.5 million, and the number of hotel rooms on the island nearly doubled (Pérez-López, 2002). Tourism and family remittances are now leading sources of hard currency for the Cuban government (Tamayo, 2002; Pérez-López, 2002).

The holding of American dollars by Cuban citizens was legalized in 1993 and Cubans were encouraged to spend them in previously forbidden "dollar stores," special state run shops that historically have been open only to diplomats and tourists. Dollar stores sell a variety of luxury and imported goods such as soap, shampoo, cooking oil, beer, and other groceries that are typically unavailable in the state or peso sector of the economy. As the state food distribution system became increasingly unreliable during the 1990s, dollar stores have become the primary means of procuring essential commodities (including basic foodstuffs) for many Cuban families.

Around one hundred types of craftsmen and artisans (such as bicycle repairmen, watch repairmen . . . etc.) are now allowed to be self employed. In 1993 there were about 15,000 of these "cuentapropistas" in Cuba. By 1996 this had grown to over 200,000 (Peters and Scarpaci, 1998). One of the more popular forms of self-employment became the operation of small, family run restaurants (known as *paladares*) in private homes. Paladares typically charge in American dollars, and offer a much cheaper (and better) alternative to the high prices, poor service and limited menu choices of state restaurants. A number of new sociedad anonimas have also been founded since the early 1990s to encourage tourism and investment by foreign firms. These include such groups as Gaviota, Rumbos, Cubanacan, and Cubalse. These firms engaged in a wide range of economic activities: retail stores, car rental businesses, hotel chains, import-export of various commodities such as rum and tobacco.

Instead of facilitating political liberalization, however, the Cuban government has structured privatization in ways that reinforce existing power structures, and further concentrate wealth and power in the hands of political elites (Corrales, 2004; Crabb, 2001; Suchlicki, 2000). As Corrales has described, "The [economic] reforms were carried out in a manner that enlarged the leverage of the state over society, rather than diminishing it" (2004:36). Corrales goes on to refer to these economic reforms as a type of "stealth statism," that has allowed the regime to maintain its authoritarian control despite the appearance of economic liberalization (p. 49).

Most of Cuba's privatized firms, for instance, are owned and operated by the Cuban Ministry of the Interior (also known as MININT, the internal police and state security services) or the Ministry of the Armed Forces (MINFAR). In other words, the fall of the Soviet Union has not led to demilitarization in Cuba. Instead, the Cuban armed forces and security services have been given an entrepreneurial role, and are now tasked with earning hard currency for the regime in a variety of economic endeavors. Individual Cubans who seek employment in these ventures must have strong ties to either the Communist Party, the military or the internal security forces. Foreign firms are not allowed to privately contract with individual Cubans for employment. Instead, the state decides who among its most loyal adherents (communist party militants, military leaders or other collaborators) is to be rewarded with an opportunity to earn hard currency in the privatized sectors of the economy (Corrales, 2004; Crabb, 2001).

The main holding company of the Cuban military is GAESA (Grupo de Administración Empresarial, S. A.). GAESA is operated by high ranking military officials, including Luis Alberto Rodríguez, the son-in-law of Raul Castro, Cuba's commander-in-chief. GAESA includes over ten diverse subsidiaries, such as Gaviota (a tourism corporation that operates over thirty hotels); Tecnotex (an import/export company); and Almacenes Universal (which operates a number of free trade zones) (Corrales, 2004; Eckstein, 1994; Espinosa, 2001). CIMEX remains the largest of the sociedad anonimas, and is controlled by officials in Cuba's Ministry of the Interior. CIMEX includes over forty-eight subsidiaries and twelve associated companies that operate in seventeen countries. Cimex is the parent company of Havanatour, a tourism business that has sold Cuban vacations to millions of Europeans and Canadians. Cimex also exports seafood, meat products, sugar, cigars, rum, software, and biotechnology products. It maintains its own merchant fleet in Panama that delivers Cuban goods throughout the Caribbean. Cimex is also a key backer of Cuba's Banco Financiero, a bank that operates in international stock and commodity markets (Corrales, 2004; Eckstein, 1994:70).

Privatization and the Health Sector

Privatization and the increasing participation of the Cuban military in corporate activities have led to significant impoverishment of the public health sector and sharp declines in community health and sanitation. Most urban neighborhoods in Havana and Santiago now have frequent water shortages, irregular electricity, deteriorated housing, poorly functioning sewer systems, irregular trash pickup and significant problems with insects and rodents (see Isla, 2005; Fernandez, 2000; Halperin, 1994). Municipal public health and sanitation programs suffer from acute shortages of equipment and other supplies. Pharmacies in the peso sector typically have little on their shelves other than a few bottles of vitamin tablets, or some aspirin. There are no supplies of soap, bandages, disinfectants, anti-diarrheals, disposable syringes, detergents, toothpaste, antibiotic creams, pain medications, cough drops, antifungals, or other basic health supplies available for purchase in the peso sector.

Most of these items, however, are now offered for sale on the black market, or at state-run international clinics and dollar pharmacies. In the early 1990s *Sociedad Anonimas* such as Servimed opened chains of fee-for-service clinics and pharmacies in most cities. Cuba has aggressively marketed these clinics abroad, and people all over the world are encouraged to travel to Cuba for reduced-rate medical procedures (see Feinsilver, 1993; Charatan, 2001).

Elite families (meaning those with strong military or political connections) cope with deteriorating environmental conditions by using cash to purchase necessary supplies and medications in the dollar sector of the economy, as well as privately contracting with carting services to have trash removed, using surplus cooking fuel to boil their drinking water, and using political connections to secure treatment in better quality hospitals. Poor (and politically disenfranchised) families, on the other hand, must live in trash-strewn neighborhoods with overflowing sewers, and frequently suffer shortages of cooking fuel that make them unable to boil their drinking water. Peso hospitals also regularly reuse glass syringes for inoculations.

The Underground Clinic

The intrusive government presence in the formal health sector, along with the relentless shortages of medical supplies has led to the formation of a dual system of health services. In my research communities in Havana and Santiago, for instance, almost no one sought medical advice from his or her official family doctor. Instead, people resolved health problems the same way they approached food shortages or bureaucratic difficulties: through *sociolismo*. Instead of consulting with their assigned health professionals, most people solicited medical advice from friends, neighbors and family members. Sometimes these individuals were health professionals, sometimes not. When formal health services were utilized, *socios* were still important in securing access to scarce medical supplies.

The importance of having reliable *socios* in the medical profession was underscored in many of the patient narratives I collected. Some individuals related harrowing stories of medical mismanagement and malpractice that were only resolved through the timely intervention of one or more well-placed *socios*. In some cases, patients could not schedule surgeries or other urgent procedures until their *socios* had been able to pilfer enough anesthetic, needles, surgical thread and medications to perform the operation. In other cases, *socios* performed bureaucratic favors, such as engineering a transfer to a more desirable hospital (such as one with air-conditioning and running water) or a more competent surgeon. Sophisticated underground trade networks existed which could supply almost any pharmaceutical drug.

Sociolismo is valuable in that it offers patients options in a system where choice is otherwise nonexistent, as well as a way to circumvent the political surveillance embedded in the formal health sector. Unfortunately, the underground economy in health services is fueled largely by theft or pilferage from the formal economy. Goods that flow into the formal health sector from the central ministry in Havana are typically stolen and resold or bartered on the black market.

These practices leave the formal health system almost an empty shell, while much of the actual business of medicine (diagnosis, treatment, and obtaining pharmaceuticals) is conducted through personal networks of *socios* using pilfered medical supplies.[7] These practices greatly impede the Cuban government's goal of maintaining social equality throughout the health care system. The informal economy is driven by a combination of generalized reciprocity and market forces: in some cases medical favors are exchanged for cash or barter, in others they are done as favor for friends and family, with the expectation that at some undefined point in the future a similar favor will be returned. Individuals with greater access to resources (such as high-ranking Party of military officials) are inevitably able to obtain much higher quality medical care than those without good connections or powerful *socios*.

These practices can also have a negative impact on population health, and make national health planning extremely difficult. Patients who obtain supplies and medications on the black market are also at risk for a host of potential complications. The informal economy is by definition unregulated, and the goods that circulate therein are uninspected and potentially adulterated. In the case of medications, illicit pharmaceuticals could very well be outdated or inappropriate for certain patients. Medicines obtained in the informal economy are also obtained and administered without a doctor's supervision, no doubt greatly increasing the possibility of negative side effects, toxicity or inappropriate dosages.

The popular reliance on the informal economy in health services in Cuba is also problematic in that it inevitably confounds researchers who seek to measure the health effects of the United States' trade embargo against Cuba (Garfield and Holtz, 2000; Garfield, 2004). It is very easy, for instance, for the Cuban government to point to the severe shortages and disarray of the formal health sector as evidence of the negative impact of the U.S. embargo (which prohibits importation of food and medicines). Without taking into account the tremendous volume of goods and services that circulate in the informal sector, however, these data are likely to be misleading.

Emerging Infectious Disease

Despite these increasing inequalities in living conditions and medical care, Cuba's national health statistics do not indicate that infectious diseases are a significant problem for the island's poor. To the contrary, rates of tuberculosis, HIV, gastrointestinal and respiratory diseases have remained dramatically lower in Cuba than in neighboring countries. In Haiti, for example, the World Health Organization has reported a TB incidence rate of approximately 319 per 100,000 population (WHO, 2004). In the Dominican Republic, the rate is approximately ninety-five per 100,000 (WHO, 2004). By comparison, Cuba's incidence rate is exceptionally low, ranging between 4.8 per 100,000 and 14.7 per 100,000 between 1991 and 1997 (Marreroa et al., 2000).

Even if Cuba's infectious disease rates are as low as contemporary MINISAP claim, some important changes have taken place in recent years in the world of microbes that are likely to pose significant health challenges for Cuba in the near future. In the 1950s when Castro took power, it was common in public health and international development to speak of a single "epidemiological transition." This referred to the demographic changes that took place once a society had effectively controlled infectious disease, and overall population mortality patterns began to shift to chronic diseases such as heart disease and cancer (see Goldschneider, 1971).

Historical evidence suggests that Cuba's epidemiological transition from infectious to chronic disease was already underway at the time of the 1959 Revolution. The militarization of the health sector in the early 1960s probably served to complete this transition, fully modernizing Cuba's mortality and demographic profiles. Over the past twenty five years, however, a number of new infectious conditions have emerged (such as HIV) throughout the world to become major contributors to adult morbidity and mortality. In some cases, global transportation networks have facilitated the spread of these "emerging infectious diseases," and in other cases medical science itself has played a role. The emergence of lethal antibiotic resistant forms of tuberculosis, strep and staph infections, for instance, can be seen as an inevitable evolutionary outcome of the widespread use (and misuse) of antibiotics over several generations (see Farmer, 1999; Garrett, 2000; Barrett et al., 1997).

Numerous epidemics of dengue fever have occurred throughout Latin America in recent years, a trend many researchers relate to lapses in mosquito control, as well as evolution of pesticide resistant strains of insects. Many strains of malaria are now resistant to pharmaceutical prophylaxis, and common insecticides are no longer effective in combating disease-carrying insects. Some scholars and activists have also approached this problem from a macro-level position, arguing that structural variables such as economic inequality, class conflict, poverty and oppression have greatly facilitated the spread of these contemporary epidemics of infectious disease, which disproportionately affect the poor (Farmer, 1999; Kim et al., 2000).

Cuba's current national health statistics do not indicate that emerging infectious diseases are a problem on the island, which still boasts of a fully "modern" mortality profile, with low infant mortality and most adult deaths occurring from chronic conditions such as heart disease, cancer or stroke. The events surrounding the 1997 epidemic of dengue fever in Santiago, however, raise a number of troubling questions about the reliability of Cuba's health reports with respect to emerging infectious disease.

During my time in Cuba, it was easy to observe that vector control and public health prevention efforts in major cities were seriously deficient. Local hospitals reused glass syringes, adequate sterilization materials or equipment was often broken or unavailable, drinking water was contaminated, cooking fuel shortages made it very difficult for people to boil drinking water, and water shortages meant that in some neighborhoods people had to store water in their homes in large barrels that bred clouds of mosquitoes.

In many neighborhoods housing was dilapidated and of poor quality, insects proliferated, trash removal was haphazard, sewage periodically overflowed onto the streets. Prostitutes as young as fifteen or sixteen years competed for the affections of significantly older tourists with few precautions against sexually transmitted diseases. According to a recent report published in the *Nuevo Herald*, a number of dissident physicians in Cuba have described widespread outbreaks of infectious disease affecting children, as well ongoing government censorship and repression regarding these negative trends. One doctor recently described the situation as "extremely grave" (Isla, 2005). Other informal sources have reported increasing problems with dysentery and other waterborne diseases in recent years, as well as deliberate manipulation of mortality data to obscure negative health trends (see Rofes, 2000; CubaNet News, February 11, 2002; May 31, 2002; October 23, 2002).

Given these environmental conditions, it seems logic to assume that emerging infectious diseases are increasing in Cuba. If the government's handling of the 1997 dengue fever epidemic is any indication, however, it appears that outbreaks are being met with authoritarian repression and denial rather than aggressive health education or public health prevention measures. These tactics may temporarily preserve Cuba's favorable image as a "world medical power" (see Feinsilver, 1993) but they will likely result in major health declines once Cuba reaches its own post-socialist transition.

Notes

1. There have been a number of excellent analyses of militarization under the Castro regime. See Horowitz (2003); Walker (1993; 2003); Suchlicki (2003); Del Aguila (2003); Fernández (1989); Del Aguila (1989); Gouré (1989); Walker (1989); Espinosa (2003).

2. Arms and narcotics trafficking by the Castro regime have been documented by Booth (1996); Herzog (1987); Oppenheimer (1993); Kempe (1990; *San Diego Union* (November 21, 1991); Fernandez (1996); Eckstein (1994); and Masetti (1996).

3. At this point it bears repeating that one Marxist scholar erroneously described Cuba's infant mortality rate prior to 1959 as "one of the worst in the world" (Waitzkin, 1983).

4. These 1997 figures were taken from a MINISAP pamphlet posted on display at the Health Economic conference at the University of the Oriente.

5. Montaner (1981) has claimed that the Castro government performs medical experiments on political prisoners, but to my knowledge these allegations have not been thoroughly investigated. It is widely recognized that the regime denies medical care to political prisoners. See Berre (undated); Human Rights Watch (1999); Valladares (1986).

6. For additional information on the Castro regime's policies in the area of gender, sexuality and family, see Montaner (1981); Arenas (1991); Smith and Padula (1996); Lear (2003).

7. Reports from the former Soviet Union illustrate a strikingly similar pattern with respect to underground markets in health services. See Feshbach and Friendly (1992); Ledeneva (1998); Knaus, (1981); Garrett (2000).

11

Conclusions

This project began in 1995 with a relatively simple goal: to learn something about the first hand realities of socialist health systems before socialism becomes completely extinct. This desire coalesced into a research plan featuring an ethnographic study of Cuba's family doctor program. The specific goals of the project developed from a review of academic literature, nearly all of which described the 1959 revolution and transition to socialism in Cuba as leading to dramatic health improvements on the island as well as great innovations in clinical care. These health improvements had been described quantitatively, in the form of improved population health statistics, but never qualitatively, in the form of ethnographic interviews, participant observation or other first hand experience in Cuban health clinics. My dissertation research was intended to remedy this oversight by exploring the qualitative dimensions of Cuba's transformations in health and medicine since 1959.

The overwhelmingly positive portrayal of Cuba in the academic literature led me to anticipate a positive research experience. It was quite a shock to arrive in Havana and discover that the reality of Cuban medicine bore little resemblance to the descriptions I had read in academic journals. Or, to put it another way, there seemed to be a host of important variables excluded from mainstream research on the Cuban health care system. These included the overwhelming importance of the informal economy, the use of *socios* and *sociolismo* to satisfy basic consumer needs (including health needs), the repressive authoritarianism of the state, the lack of individual rights such as privacy and free speech, the widespread discontent and disillusionment with the socialist system (often manifest in outrageous black humor and deliberate parasitism on public resources through theft or black market activity), the disregard for public welfare and neglect of basic public health prevention measures on the part of government authorities, the chilling Cold War militarism, xenophobia and anti-Americanism displayed by the regime, and the widespread vice and corruption (including prostitution and sex tourism) that have resulted from recent privatization of the economy.

Any residual idealism I might have had about the Cuban health care system quickly evaporated once I discovered the Cuban government was trying to hide a major epidemic of dengue fever during my stay in Santiago. The repression and mismanagement of this epidemic, as well as my negative experiences as a patient led me to reject nearly all of the academic literature that originally framed my dissertation research proposal. The arrest and imprisonment of Dr. Desi Mendoza (the dissident physician who broke the story of the dengue epidemic to the international media) on charges of "disseminating counterrevolutionary propaganda" reinforced my suspicion that the Castro regime's early enthusiasm for improving health and medicine has largely been replaced by censorship and manipulation of health data. Unfortunately, the constraints Cuba places on foreign researchers made it impossible to empirically investigate these less favorable aspects of health care.

History Revisited

One avenue of further research that did remain open (and that could be conducted in the United States) was archival research. Early historical documents I discovered in Santiago led me to suspect that in addition to manipulating health data of the present, the Castro regime has also sought to manipulate the health data of past in order to magnify its own contribution to Cuba's favorable mortality profile. This suspicion led to a new research project investigating health conditions in Cuba during the early part of the twentieth century. Research in archival collections in the United States revealed a number of discrepancies between contemporary representations of Cuba's health history, and the way these events were described in original documents.

The relationship between U.S. policies and health trends on the island, for instance, appears to have been very different from dependency model used by many contemporary scholars. Most of the assumptions medical anthropologists have made about Cuba's "pre-revolutionary" health trends have been based on historical correlations linking the increase in U.S. investment in Cuba with the increasing incidence of U.S. political and military intervention. The implicit assumption has been that U.S. political muscle, in the form of military occupations, was used to pave the way for American capitalists to take control of Cuba's resources. This expansion of foreign capital is portrayed as the ultimate cause of Cuba's impoverishment, underdevelopment and poor health conditions prior to 1959 (see Baer, 1989; Elling, 1989; Singer and Baer, 1989; Singer and Baer, 1995; Singer, Baer and Lazarus, 1990; Waitzkin, 1983; Waitzkin and Britt, 1989).

Historical documents portray these events very differently. According to observers at the time, U.S. political and military interventions between 1898 and 1933 were motivated in part by a desire to prop up Cuba's failing public sector (including its health and sanitation infrastructure), not solely to coerce Cuban politicians into governing in the interests of foreign capital. At least part of the United States' goal in intruding into Cuban politics was to subdue political violence, and maintain oversight over sanitation programs, as exemplified by Article Five of the Platt Amendment. Unfortunately, the effects of this amendment were often the opposite of its intended purpose. The Platt Amendment hopelessly politicized health in Cuba and resulted in generations of *caudillo*-driven health propaganda rather than genuine national investment in public health prevention efforts.

U.S. interventions in Cuba were also motivated by a certain degree of self-interest—infectious diseases in Cuba frequently traveled by steamship to port cities in the southern U.S. Racism also played a role. Political leaders in the United States subscribed to a racist belief that "Latin" republics could not maintain adequate standards of sanitation. Regardless of whether the motives were selfish or altruistic, however, the impact of the U.S. military occupations in the area of health and disease was generally positive.

The vocabulary of Marxism and dependency theory also effectively erases many of the historical continuities between the Castro regime and its predecessors. In the Marxist model, "socialist" and "capitalist" are presented as mutually exclusive categories. These linguistic distortions have led many scholars to overlook the "socialist" aspects of Castro's predecessors (the state came to control increasingly large sectors of the economy from the 1930s to the 1950s) in favor of a model that portrays all previous leaders as tools of foreign capital. Correspondingly, many contemporary scholars have ignored the "capitalist" elements of Castro's regime (integration into global markets and privatization of key sectors of the economy) in favor of a model that portrays the Cuban economy as largely egalitarian and state-controlled.

The forgotten history of the 1959 revolution, of course, reveals that Fidel Castro's rise to power paralleled that of almost every other Cuban leader in the twentieth century: he was originally part of an exile coalition made up of the combined forces of all groups opposed to the existing regime; he collaborated with North American organized crime groups to secure weapons and financial backing for his insurrectionary movement, and he aggressively lobbied the United States to intervene and oust the existing leader (Batista) on humanitarian grounds. Once in power he became violently opposed to any U.S. intervention in Cuba, sought to take sole power and exclude rival revolutionary groups from the new government. When he became established as the sole ruler, he then repeated (or even intensified) many of the abuses of his predecessors: aggressive militarization, jailing or forcing political opposition groups into exile, vastly increasing the size and scope of the public sector and (in recent years) rewarding political followers with specialized opportunities to earn capital in the newly privatized sectors of the economy.

Most conventional accounts within medical anthropology overlook these continuities in favor of reiterating the Castro regime's own historical mythology: Fidel Castro is portrayed as the secular savior of Cuba, and the 1959 revolution is described as the final realization of José Martí's dream of *Cuba Libre*. In a 1971 speech recorded by a visiting American student, Castro himself described the Revolution in these rather apocalyptic terms,

> History to this time he [Fidel] told us, has really been prehistory. It has been barbarous, cruel and death-oriented. We are now entering into the era of true human history—the New Man. He spoke of massive changeover in the nature of the world. . . . And he stood there and explained to us how the entire world would rise up against the old, dead order and create an entire, radically new life for man . . . Imperialism, capitalism, all that is old and decaying will surely lose. Our task is to make ourselves ready and

able to build from those ruins a truly humane society—void of the anarchy and insanity that traditionally follow the destruction of empires. I firmly believe now that we must 'learn communism' as Lenin said. It is not just an economic theory, but the basis on which this world *must* move toward a new society (quoted in Levinson and Brightman, 1971:344).

Time and space have even been reconfigured in Cuba to be in accordance with this historical mythology. Chronological time is now reckoned not only by the regular calendar but also the revolutionary calendar. The year 1999, for instance, is also referred to as "year 40 of the glorious revolution" in all government publications and media sources. Chronological time before 1959 is correspondingly characterized as an undifferentiated "pre-revolutionary era" characterized by uniform suffering and oppression. The specifics of these years have largely been forgotten.

This historical revisionism is manifest spatially as well. Havana is dotted with historical monuments and statues erected to commemorate key leaders or other important events in the twentieth century. President José Miguel Gómez erected a massive monument to himself near the University of Havana in the early 1900s. Presidents Zayas and Menocal named parks and streets after themselves, and in Santiago a park was built on San Juan Hill to commemorate Teddy Roosevelt and the Rough Riders. All of these historical and cultural landmarks have either been deliberately stripped of identifiers or allowed to decay into meaninglessness by the Castro regime. The Gomez monument is now unmarked and littered with trash and graffiti. The streets and parks near the capitol have been renamed. And in Santiago the plaques have been completely removed from the statues of the Rough Riders, who stand as faceless sentinels on San Juan Hill.

In contrast, the Castro regime has erected numerous monuments and statues to José Marti, Antonio Maceo and other Cuban heroes of the War of Independence against Spain, juxtaposed together with memorials to Che Guevara and other leaders of the 1959 Revolution. This spatial linking of the independence movement against Spain with contemporary icons of the 1959 Revolution, combined with the deliberate erasure and neglect of memorials to all other twentieth century leaders provides a powerful visual counterpoint to the government's rhetoric.

One key difference that has distinguished the Castro regime from its predecessors was the substitution of a culture of civic honesty for the former culture of graft and patronage that previously characterized the public sector. This accomplishment, combined with the aggressive militarization of the health sector that took place in the early 1960s most likely did lead to a number of positive improvements in health conditions on the island. The expansion of health services to previously under served areas of the country was also a significant accomplishment. It is difficult to ascertain the true magnitude of health improvement brought about by these developments, since (like earlier *caudillo* regimes) the Castro government has sought to discredit its rivals by releasing significant amounts of distorted health data. Recent events would seem to imply that there has been considerable decline in public health prevention and in the quality of clinical medicine in recent years.

Political Capitalism

One of the key goals of presenting this revisionist history has been to argue that a Weberian, rather than a Marxist model of political economy, offers more analytical power in making sense of Cuba's twentieth century health trends. *Caudillos* are political capitalists, who use personalistic armies to seize government power as a spoils system. Their followers are rewarded with patronage positions or other opportunities to acquire wealth, such as gambling or smuggling concessions in the informal economy. Opponents of *caudillo* regimes, on the other hand, are often excluded from meaningful participation in both formal and informal sectors of the economy. Personalistic armies and public officials are deployed to abet the capital accumulation of the loyal and to attack the capital of the opposition. Opposition leaders respond to these challenges with violence, and the resulting conflicts often lead to destructive cycles of political-economic decline. As Stephen Krasner has described, failed (or failing) states typically exhibit a common set of problems,

> In such [failed] states, infrastructure deteriorates; corruption is widespread; borders are unregulated; gross domestic product is declining or stagnant; crime is rampant; and the national currency is not widely accepted. Armed groups operate within the state's boundaries but outside the control of the government. . . . Authority may be exercised by local entities in other parts of the country, or by no one at all . . . Decisions affecting the distribution

of wealth are based on personal connections rather than bureaucratic regulations or the rule of law (2004:91–92).

These characteristics aptly describe political and economic conditions in Cuba for many years prior to 1959. Political violence and insurrections erupted frequently, and at times entire provinces fell under the control of armed rebel bands that extorted informal "taxes" from local businesses and foreign capitalists. The dividing line between rebel groups and gangsters in Cuba was also poorly defined: many of Cuba's most famous revolutionaries financed their activities through deals with North American and Canadian organized crime groups. Rebels smuggled narcotics or other contraband to gangsters, who in turn supplied arms and explosives. If the rebels were successful (as they were in 1933 and 1959) the gangsters were rewarded with lucrative gambling and smuggling concessions inside Cuba. The tremendous wealth accumulated by Cuban politicians and their associates in organized crime inevitably stimulated the formation of new rebel groups and new insurrectionary movements.

Political Capitalism and Health

Political capitalism and *caudillismo* both have negative implications for health. The personalism and corruption of *caudillo* rule means that state health programs are underfunded and disorganized. The chronic instability and violence of *caudillo* regimes also destabilizes the natural environment in ways that facilitate outbreaks of infectious diseases. Without an adequate public health infrastructure, epidemics inevitably result. The high rates of typhoid that prevailed in Cuba in the 1940s, for instance, resulted from the failure of the state to supply clean drinking water to the urban population. This failure was not due to lack of funds, but to the wholesale diversion of Ministry of Health dollars into private hands. As medical technology advanced over the course of the twentieth century, private sector medicine in Cuba became equipped to contain (though not prevent) many of these disease outbreaks. The development of a relatively safe, effective typhoid vaccine in the 1950s, for instance, proved to be a much more effective means to combat typhoid outbreaks in Cuba than lobbying the corrupt *caudillo*-government to construct a new waterworks for the population of Havana. The increased availability of pesticides such as DDT also had a significant impact on rates of malaria in many parts of the developing world during this time. During this time innovative mutualist societies such as the Centro Gallego and the Centro Austuriano were able to provide access to quality clinical medicine for thousands of working class Cubans at low cost.

As a result of these improvements in medical technology, and the widespread availability of clinical medicine in Cuba through the 1940s and 1950s, health indicators began to show some improvements despite the inability of the public sector to adequately control disease vectors. Chronic illnesses such as heart disease and cancer began to replace infectious diseases as leading causes of death, and the infant mortality rate dropped to a level that was quite low for Latin America at this time. The failures of the public sector, however, probably prevented Cuba from fully realizing a "modern" mortality profile. As long as drinking water remained contaminated, and with so many rural families were marginally nourished, infectious diseases such as gastritis and enteritis continued to be major causes of death in the 1950s.

Afterwards: Rejecting Marxism

Despite the weaknesses of the Marxist and dependency models in explaining Cuba's twentieth century health trends, they have shown remarkable staying power in academia. The Castro regime's portrayal of the Spanish-American War and U.S. imperialism during the Platt era have become routinely accepted and reproduced in mainstream Latin American Studies scholarship. Events or individuals that do not fit the Marxist model have remained unexamined or been allowed to fade from historical memory.

In my own case, first hand experience with the discrepancies between rhetoric and reality in Cuba made rejecting the Marxist model relatively straightforward. After a few months on the island, Marx's ideal of socialism seemed like an obsolete fantasy that explained nothing about the realities of everyday life. If popular discourse and subterranean humor are any indication, many Cubans (and Russians, and eastern Europeans—see Eisenstadt, 1992; Gleason, 1997; Kolakowski, 1992; Malia, 1994; Havel, 1999; Ries, 1997) share my skepticism. Given the unavoidable chasm that prevails between everyday reality and the Marxist ideal in Cuba, the continued orthodoxy of Marxist theory in medical anthropology and Latin American studies scholarship on Cuba is troubling. Why have anthropologists so routinely accepted Cuban government communiqués as representative of "the native's point of view" in their scholarship on Cuba? Why have the subaltern voices of dissidents remained excluded from the writings of medical anthropologists and public health researchers? Are historical events and cultural memories continually "misshapen" by the collective ideological biases of professional historians and other academics, as has been charged by Harvey Klehr and John Haynes (see Haynes and Klehr, 2003)?

Any thorough investigation of these questions would be far beyond the scope of this book. My goal in posing them is simply to encourage other scholars to broaden their research agendas and consider alternative theoretical models with respect to understanding twentieth century patterns of health and disease in Latin America and the Caribbean. Even a casual review of history reveals that *caudillismo*, corruption, and political instability have been common themes throughout the region. The relationship between these political-economic variables and epidemics of infectious disease merits further exploration.

Bibliography

Acosta, Dalia (1997) Cuba: Health Still a Jewel in Castro's Crown. *InterPress News Service*, April 9.

Adler, Patricia and Adler, Peter (1987) *Membership Roles in Field Research.* Newbury Park, CA: Sage Publications.

Aguilar, Louis (1972) *Cuba 1933: Prologue to Revolution.* Ithaca, NY: Cornell University Press.

Alarcón de Quesada, Ricardo (1997) This People will Never be Enslaved, nor will Cuba be Converted into a U.S. Colony. Speech before the National Assembly of People's Power, reprinted in *Granma International*, February 19.

Alexander, Robert (1969) *Communism in Latin America.* New Brunswick, NJ: Rutgers University Press.

Alibek, Ken (1999) *Biohazard.* New York: Random House.

Alvarez del Real, Evelio (1942) *Patrias Opacas y Caudillos Fulgurantes.* Havana: La Veronica.

Ameringer, Charles (1996) *The Caribbean Legion: Patriots, Politicians, Soldiers of Fortune, 1946–1950.* University Park, PA: Pennsylvania State University Press.

Amnesty International (2000) *Cuba: Short Term Detention and Harassment of Dissidents.* New York: Amnesty International.

Andreski, Stanislav (1966) *Parasitism and Subversion: The Case of Latin America.* New York: Random House.

Arenas, Reinaldo (1994) *The Assault.* New York: Penguin Books.

Arenas, Reinaldo (1993) *Before Night Falls.* New York: Viking Press.

Aron, Raymond (1957) *The Opium of the Intellectuals.* Garden City: Doubleday and Co.

Baer, Hans (1989) Towards a Critical Medical Anthropology of Health Related Issues in Socialist-Oriented Countries. *Medical Anthropology*, 11:181–193.

Baer, Hans (1990). The Possibilities and Dilemmas of building Bridges Between Critical Medical Anthropology and Clinical Anthropology: A Discussion. *Social Science and Medicine* 30(9): 1011–1013.

Baer, Hans, Singer, Merrill and Johnsen, John (1986) Toward a Critical Medical Anthropology. *Social Science and Medicine*, 23(2):95–98.

Bahro, Rudolf (1978) *The Alternative in Eastern Europe.* London: Verso.

Bangs, John Kedrick (1902) *Uncle Sam, Trustee.* New York: Riggs Publishing.

Barnet, Enrique (1905) *La Sanidad de Cuba.* La Habana: Imprente Mercantil Teniente Rey.

237

Barnet, E.B. (1913) *Consideraciones sobre el estado sanitario de Cuba.* La Habana: Academia de Ciencias Médicas.

Barnet, Enrique (1914) *Conversaciones del Doctor.* La Habana.

Barrett, Ronald, Kuzawa, Christopher, McDade, Thomas and Armelagos, George (1998) Emerging and Re-Emerging Infectious Diseases: The Third Epidemiologic Transition. *Annual Review of Anthropology,* 27:247–271.

Batista Fulgencio (1962) *Cuba Betrayed.* New York: Vantage Press.

Batista, Fulgencio (1964) *The Growth and Decline of the Cuban Republic.* New York: Devin Adair.

Beals, Carlton (1934) *The Crime of Cuba.* Philadelphia, PA: J. Lippincott.

Benjamin, Jules (1974) *The United States and Cuba: Hegemony and Dependent Development, 1880–1934.* Pittsburgh, PA: University of Pittsburgh Press.

Benjamin, Jules (1990) *The United States and the Origins of the Cuban Revolution: An Empire of Liberty in an Age of National Liberation.* Princeton, NJ: Princeton University Press.

Berger, Peter (1974) *Pyramids of Sacrifice: Political Ethics and Social Change.* New York: Basic Books.

Berger, Peter (1977a) The Socialist Myth. In, *Facing up to Modernity: Excursions in Society, Politics and Religion.* New York: Basic Books, pp. 56–69.

Berger, Peter (1977b) Toward a Critique of Modernity. In, *Facing up to Modernity: Excursions in Society, Politics and Religion.* New York: Basic Books, pp. 70–80.

Berger, Peter (1986) *The Capitalist Revolution: Fifty Propositions about Prosperity, Equality and Liberty.* New York: Basic Books.

Berger, Peter, Berger Brigitte and Kellner, Hansfried (1973) *The Homeless Mind: Modernization and Consciousness.* Random House: New York.

Berman, Harold (1953) *The Russians In Focus.* Boston, MA: Little, Brown and Company.

Berman, Harold (1963) *Justice in the U.S.S.R.: An Interpretation of Soviet Law.* Cambridge: Harvard University Press.

Berre, Rosa (undated) Repression Against Civil Society. In, Repression in Cuba: A Battle Against the People. http://www.cubanet.org/cubanews.html.

Betancourt, Ernesto (1982) *Fidel Castro and the Bankers: Mortgaging of a Revolution.* Washington, DC: Cuban American National Foundation.

Betancourt, Ernesto (1991) *Revolutionary Strategy: A Handbook for Practitioners.* New Brunswick, NJ: Transaction Press.

Betancourt, Ernesto (2001) Economic Organizations and Post-Castro Cuba. In, *Cuban Communism,* 11th Edition, Irving Louis Horowitz, (Ed.). New Brunswick: Transaction Press, pp. 210–221.

Blackburn, Robin (1963) Prologue to the Cuban Revolution. *New Left Review,* 21(4):52–91.

Blasier, Cole (1985) *The Hovering Giant: U.S. Responses to Revolutionary Change in Latin America, 1910–1985.* Pittsburgh, PA: University of Pittsburgh Press.

Blackburn, Robin (1963) Prologue to the Cuban Revolution. *New Left Review,* 21(4):52–91.

Blas Roca (1961) *Medico Cubano, Cual es tu Porvenir.* Habana: Imprenta Nacional de Cuba.

Bloch, Sidney and Reddaway, Peter (1984) *Soviet Psychiatric Abuse: The Shadow over World Psychiatry*. London: Victor Gollancz.

Boggs, James and Boggs, Grace Lee (1974) *Revolution and Evolution in the Twentieth Century*. New York: Monthly Review Press.

Bonsal, Steven (1896) "The Real Condition of Cuba." Speech before the U.S. Senate.

Bonsal, Stephen (1912) *The American Mediterranean*. New York: Moffett, Yard and Co.

Booth, Martin (1996) *Opium: A History*. New York: St. Martin's Press.

Bradbury, Ray (1965[1945]) Skeleton. In, *Vintage Bradbury*. New York: Vintage Books, pp. 179–196.

Brady, Rose (1999) *Kapitalizm: Russia's Struggle to Free Its Economy*. New Haven, CT: Yale University Press.

British Medical Association (1992) *Medicine Betrayed: The Participation of Doctors in Human Rights Abuses*. London: Zed Press.

Brooke, John (1899) Annual Report of U.S. Army Commanding the Division of Cuba. Havana.

Brown, Charles and Lago, Armando (1991) *The Politics of Psychiatry in Revolutionary Cuba*. New Brunswick, NJ: Transaction Publishers.

Buber, Martin (1996 [1950] *Paths in Utopia*. Syracuse: Syracuse University Press.

Bunck, Julie (2003) Market-Oriented Marxism: Post-Cold War Transition in Cuba and Vietnam. In, *Cuban Communism*, 11th Edition, Irving Louis Horowitz and Jaime Suchlicki, (Eds.) New Brunswick, NJ: Transaction Press, pp. 154–175.

Burr, C. (1997) Assessing Cuba's Approach to Contain AIDS and HIV. *The Lancet*, 350:647.

Brzezinski, Zbigniew (1989) *The Grand Failure: The Birth and Death of Communism in the Twentieth Century*. New York: Charles Scribner's Sons.

CDR (1964) *El MINISAP y los CDR en Las Tareas de Salud*. La Habana.

CDR (1966) *Guia de Sectoristas*. La Habana.

Cabrera-Infante, Guillermo (1994) *Mea Cuba*. London: Faber and Faber.

Caldwell, John (1993) Health Transition: The Cultural, Social and Behavioral Determinants of Health in the Third World. Social Science and Medicine, 36(2):125–135.

Callari. Antonio, Cullenberg, Stephen and Biewener, Carole (1996) Introduction. In, *Marxism in the Postmodern Age: Confronting the New World Order*. Callari, Cullenberg and Biewener, (Eds.) New York: Guilford Press, pp. 1–12.

Castellanos, Augustín (1962a) *La Medicina en Cuba Hoy*. Unpublished manuscript. Cuban Exile Medical Association. University of Miami Archives.

Castellanos, Augustín (1962b) *La Gran Tragedia de la Salud en Cuba*. Unpublished manuscript. Cuban Exile Medical Association. University of Miami Archives.

Castellanos, Augustín (1963) *La Terrible Crisis de la Medicina en La Cuba Castrista*. Unpublished Manuscript. Cuban Exile Medical Association. University of Miami Archives.

Castro Ruz, Fidel (1982) Speech at the 2nd Congress of the CDRs, October 24, 1981. In, Castro, *Fidel Speeches at Three Congresses*. Havana: Editoria Politica.

Castro Ruz, Fidel (1986[1989]) Renewal or Death. Speech before the Third Party Congress, Havana Cuba, Febrary 7, 1986. Reprinted in *The Black Scholar*, 20(5–6):7.

Castro Ruz, Fidel (1997a) The More we are Harassed, the More our Strength, our Hatred of Injustice and our Love for Socialism will Grow. Speech commemorating the 40th anniversary of the assault of the presidential palace and the takeover of Radio Reloj, reprinted in *Granma Internacional*, April 2.

Castro Ruz, Fidel (2005) Speech given at the first graduation of the Latin American School of Medicine.

Castro Ruz, Raul (1997b) A Cuba Podrán Tratar de Destruirla, pero Nadie dude que Jamás Podrán Conquistarla. Speech commemorating the 44th anniversary of the assualt on the Moncada Barracks, reprinted in *Granma*, March 29.

Chapman, Charles (1927) *A History of the Cuban Republic*. New York: Macmillan and Co.

Chartaran, Fred (2001) Foreigners Flock to Cuba for Medical Care. *East West Journal of Medicine*, 175:81.

Chesnais, Jean-Claude (1992) *The Demographic Transition: Stages, Patterns and Economic Implications*. Oxford: Clarendon Press.

Chevalier, Francois (1965) The Roots of Personalism. In, *Dictatorship in Spanish America*, Hammill, Hugh, (Ed.). New York: Afred A. Knopf, pp. 35–51.

Chomsky, Aviva (2000) The Threat of a Good Example: Health and Revolution in Cuba. In, *Dying for Growth: Global Inequality and the Health of the Poor*. Monroe, ME: Common Courage Press, pp. 331–358.

Chomsky, Noam (1994) Introduction. In, Farmer, Paul, *The Uses of Haiti*. Monroe, ME: Common Courage Press, pp. 13–44.

Cirules, Enrique (2003) *The Mafia in Havana*. Melbourne, Australia: Ocean Press.

Clark, William (1898) *Commercial Cuba: A Book for Businessmen*. New York: Scribners.

Clifford, James (2002) *The Predicament of Culture*. Boston, MA: Harvard University Press.

Cockerham, William (1999) *Health and Social Change in Russia and Eastern Europe*. New York: Routledge.

Cole, Johnetta (1979) *Race to Equality: The Impact of the Cuban Revolution on Racism*. La Habana.

Cole, Johnetta (1988) Women in Cuba: The Revolution within the Revolution. In, *Anthropology for the Nineties*, Johnetta B. Cole, (Ed.)., New York: The Free Press, pp. 532–545.

Commission on Cuban Affairs (1935) *Problems of the New Cuba*. New York: Foreign Policy Association.

Corbett, Ben (2002) *This is Cuba: An Outlaw Culture Survives*. Boulder, CO: Westview Press.

Cordova, Efren and Mourie, Eduardo García (2001) Labor Conditions in Revolutionary Cuba. In, *Cuban Communism*, 11th Edition, Irving Louis Horowitz, (Ed.). New Brunswick, NJ: Transaction Press, pp. 122–133.

Corrales, Javier (2004) The Gatekeeper State: Limited Economic Reforms and Regime Survival in Cuba, 1989–2002. *Latin American Research Review*, 39(2):36–65.

Crabb, Mary Katherine (1998) *Decline of the State, Growth of the Nation: Nationalism and Caudillo Politics in Early Republican Cuba*. Paper presented at the Bastards of Imperialism Conference, Stanford University, Stanford, CA.

Crabb, Mary Katherine (2001) The Political Economy of Caudillismo: A Critique of Recent Economic Reforms in Cuba. In, *Cuban Communism,* Horowitz, Irving Louis and Suchlicki, Jaime, (Eds.) New Brunswick: Transaction Press

The Cuban Report (1964) *Illness of Infants in Cuba in 1963.* Miami: Directorio Revolucionario Estudiantil.

Cuban Information Bureau (1931) *Ambassader Guggenheim and the Cuban Revolt.* Washington, DC: Cuban Information Bureau.

DRE (1964) Illness of Infants in Cuba in 1963. *The Cuban Report.* Miami: Cuban Student Directorate.

Daniels, Anthony (1991) *Utopias Elsewhere: Journeys in a Vanishing World.* New York: Crown Publishers.

Danielson, Ross (1977) Cuban Health Care in Process: Models and Morality in the Early Revolution: In, *Topias and Utopias in Health,* Ingram, Stanely and Thomas, Anthony, (Eds.) The Hague: Mouton Publishers, pp. 307–333.

Danielson, Ross (1979) *Cuban Medicine.* New Brunswick: Transaction Books.

Danielson, Ross (1981) Medicine in the Community: the Ideology and Substsance of Community Medicine in Socialist Cuba. *Social Science and Medicine,* 15C:239–247.

Davis, Christopher (1989) The Soviet Health Care System: A National Health Service in a Socialist Society. In, *Success and Crisis in National Health systems: A Comparative Approach,* Mark Field, (Ed.). Pp. 233–264.

Deacon, Bob (1984) Medical Care and Health under State Socialism. *International Journal of Health Services,* 14(3):453–480.

Debray, Regis (1967) *Revolution in the Revolution.* New York: Grove Press.

De Brun, Suzanne and Elling, Ray (1987) Cuba and the Phillipines: Contrasting Cases in World-System Analysis. *International Journal of Health Services,* 17(4):681–701.

DeCosse, Susan (1999*) Cuba's Repressive Machinery: Human Rights Forty Years after the Revolution.* New York: Human Rights Watch.

Del Aguila, Juan (1989) The Changing Character of Cuba's Armed Forces. In, *The Cuban Military Under Castro,* Jaime Suchlicki, (Ed.). Miami, FL: University of Miami North-South Center, pp. 27–57.

Del Aguila, Juan (2003) The Cuban Armed Forces: Changing Roles, Continued Loyalties. In, *Cuban Communism,* 11th Edition, Irving Horowitz and Jaime Suchlicki, (Eds.). New Brunswick, NJ: Transaction Press, pp. 415–427.

Del Aguila, Juan (1994a) *Cuba: Dilemmas of a Revolution.* Boulder, CO: Westview Press.

Del Aguila, Juan (1994b) The Party, the Fourth Congress, and the Process of Counterreform. In, *Cuba at the Crossroads: Politics and Economics after the Fourth Party Congress,* Perez-Lopez, (Ed.). Gainesville, Fl: University of Florida Press

De la Campa, Román (1997) Investing in Cuba. *Dissent,* 44(3):24–25.

DeYoung, Karen (2000) "Kidnapped" Cuban Defectors Disappear in Africa. *Washington Post.* June 7.

Diaz-Briquets, Sergio (1983) *The Health Revolution in Cuba.* Austin, TX: University of Texas Press.

Diaz-Briquets, Sergio (1986) How to Figure out Cuba: Development, Ideology, Mortality. *Caribbean Review,* 15(2):8–11, 39–42.

Djilas, Milovan (1998) *Fall of the New Class: A History of Communism's Self-Destruction*. New York: A.A. Knopf.

Dominguez, Nancy (1987) *Higiene Social y Organizacion de la Salud*. Havana: MINISAP.

Draper, Theodore (1962) *Castro's Revolution: Myths and Realities*. New York: Praeger.

Draper, Theodore (1964) *Castroism: Theory and Practice*. New York: Praeger.

Dresang, L.T. Brebick, L., Murray, D. et al. (2005) Family Medicine in Cuba: Community-Oriented Primary Care and Complementary Alternative Medicine. *Journal of the American Board of Family Practice*, 18(4):297–303.

Duberman, Martin (1975) The Cuban Revolution and Western Intellctuals. In, *The New Cuba: Paradoxes and Potentials,*. Radosh, Ronald, (Ed.). New York: William Morrow, pp. 35–55.

Dubois, Jules (1959) *Fidel Castro: Rebel, Liberator or Dictator*. Indianapolis: Bobbs-Merrill.

Dubos, Rene (1959) *Mirage of Health: Utopias, Progress and Biological Change*. New York: Harper and Brothers.

Dumont, Rene (1974) *Cuba—Is it Socialist?* New York: Deutch.

Dutschke, Rudi (1969) On Anti-Authoritarianism. In, *The New Left Reader*, Carl Oglesby, (Ed.). New York: Grove Press, pp. 243–254.

Eberstadt, Nicholas (1986) Did Fidel Fudge the Figures? *Caribbean Review*, 15(2):5–7, 37–38.

Eckstein, Susan (1994) *Back from the Future: Cuba under Castro*. Princeton, NJ: Princeton University Press.

Eckstein, Susan (1997) The Limits of Socialism in a Capitalist World Economy: Cuba Since the Collapse of the Soviet Block. In, *Toward a New Cuba: Legacies of a Revolution*, Centeno, Miguel and Font, Mauricio, (Eds.), Boulder, CO: Lynn Rienner, pp. 135–150.

Edwards, Jorge (1993) *Persona non Grata*. New York: Paragon House.

Eisenstadt, S.N. (1992) The Breakdown of Communist Regime and the Vicissitudes of Modernity. *Daedelus*, 121:21–42.

Elling, Ray (1989) Is Socialism Bad for your Health? Cuba and the Phillipines: A Cross-National Study of Health Systems. *Medical Anthropology*, 11:127–150.

Engle, Margarita (1993) *Singing to Cuba*. Houston, TX: Arte Publico Press.

Enzenberger, Hans Magnus (1975) Portrait of a Party: Prehistory, Structure and Ideology of the PCC. In, *The New Cuba: Paradoxes and Potentials*, Radosh, Ronald, (Ed.). New York: William Morrow, pp. 102–137.

Ernst, Morris and Loth, David (1952) *Report on the American Communist*. New York: Henry Holt.

Escalante, Fabián (1995) *The Secret War: CIA Covert Operations Against Cuba, 1959–1962*. Melbourne: Ocean Press.

Espinosa, Juan-Carlos (2003) Vanguard of the State: The Cuban Armed Forces in Transition. In, *Cuban Communism*, 11th Edition, Irving Horowitz and Jaime Suchlicki, (Eds.) New Brunswick, NJ: Transaction Press, pp. 366–387.

Ewald, Paul (1994) *The Evolution of Infectious Disease*. Oxford: Oxford University Press.

Exposito, Cesar Rodriguez (1947) *Dr. Juan Guiteras*. Havana: Editorial Cubanacan.

Fairchild, Amy and Oppenheimer, Gerald (1998) Public Health Nihilism vs. Pragmatism: History, Politics and the Control of Tuberculosis. *American Journal of Public Health*, 88(7):1105–1117.

Falk, Pamela (1987) Cuba in Africa. *Foreign Affairs*, 65(5):

Fanon, Franz (1969) Algeria Unveiled. In, *The New Left Reader*, Carl Oglesby, (Ed.). New York: Grove Press, pp. 161–185.

Farmer, Paul (1994) *The Uses of Haiti.* Monroe, ME: Common Courage Press.

Farmer, Paul (1999) *Infections and Inequalities: The Modern Plagues.* Berkeley, CA: University of California Press.

Farmer, Paul (2003) *Pathologies of Power: Health, Human Rights and the New War on the Poor.* Berkeley, CA: University of California Press.

Farmer, Paul and Bertrand, Didi (2000) Hypocrisies of Development and the Health of the Haitian Poor. In, *Dying for Growth: Global Inequality and the Health of the Poor*, Kim, Jim Yong et al., (Eds.) Monroe, Maine: Common Courage Press, pp. 65–90.

Feinsilver, Julie (1993) *Healing the Masses: Cuban Health Politics at Home and Abroad.* Berkeley, CA: University of California Press.

Fergusson, Erna (1946) *Cuba.* New York: Alfred Knopf.

Fernandez, Alina (1997) *Castro's Daughter: An Exile's Memory of Cuba.* New York: St. Martin's Press.

Fernández, Damián (1989) Historical Background: Achievements, Failures and Prospects. In, *The Cuban Military Under Castro*, Jaime Suchlicki, (Ed.). Miami, FL: University of Miami North-South Center, pp. 4–24.

Ferández, Isabel Holgado (2000) *No es Fácil! Mujeres Cubanas y la Crisis Revolucionaria.* Barcelona: Editorial Icaria.

Fernandez, Francisco (1930) The Present Status of the Practice of Medicine and Sanitation in Cuba. *Southern Medical Journal*, 23(1):6–8.

Fernandez, Wilfredo (1916) *Discurso Pronunciado en la Camara de Representantes en la Sesion del dia 19 de Junio de 1916.* La Habana: Imprenta y Papelaria de Rambla.

Ferrell, Jeff (1998) Criminological Vershtehen. In, *Ethnography at the Edge: Crime, Deviance and Field Research*, Jeff Ferrell and Mark Hamm, (Eds.) Boston, MA: Northeastern University Press, pp. 20–42.

Feshbach, Murray and Friendly, Alfred (1992) *Ecocide in the U.S.S.R.: Health and Nature under Seige.* New York: Basic Books.

Field, Mark (1989) Introduction. In, *Success and Crisis In National Health Systems : a comparative approach.* Mark G. Field, (Ed.). New York : Routledge.

Figureas, Francisco (1906) *La Intervención y su Politica.* La Habana.

Fituni, Leonid (1995) The Collapse of the Socialist State: Angola and the Soviet Union. In, Zartman, William, (Ed.). *Collapsed States: The Disintegration and Restoration of Legitimate Authority.* Boulder, CO: Lynne Reinner, pp. 143–156.

Fitzpatrick, Sheila (1999) *Everyday Stalinism.* Oxford: Oxford University Press.

Forman, James (1972) *Socialism: Its Theoretical Roots and Present-Day Development.* New York: Dell Books.

Franck, Harry (1920) *Roaming Through the West Indies.* New York: Blue Ribbon Books.

Franco, Victor (1963) *The Morning After: A French Journalist's Impression of Cuba under Castro.* New York.

Franqui, Carlos (1984) *Family Portrait with Fidel.* New York: Random House.

Friedrich, Carl and Brzezinski, Zbigniew (1965 [1956]) *Totalitarian Dictatorship and Autocracy.* New York: Frederick A. Praeger.

Frimpong-Ansah, Jonathan (1992) *The Vampire State in Africa: The Political Economy of Decline in Ghana.* Trenton, NJ: Africa World Press.

Galíndez, Jesús (1965) A Report on Santo Domingo. In, *Dictatorship in Spanish America,* Hamill, Hugh, (Ed.). New York: Alfred A. Knopf, pp. 174–187.

Garfield, Richard (2004) Health Care in Cuba and the Manipulation of Humanitarian Imperatives. *The Lancet,* 364:1007.

Garfield, Richard and Holtz, Timothy (2000) Health System reforms in Cuba in the 1990s. In, *Healthcare Reform and Poverty in Latin America,* Lloyd-Sherlock, Peter, (Ed.). London: Institute of Latin American Studies, pp. 112–127.

Garrett, Laurie (1994) *The Coming Plague: Newly Emerging Diseases in a World Out of Balance.* New York: Penguin Books.

Garrett, Laurie (2000) *Betrayal of Trust: The Collapse of Global Public Health.* New York: Hyperion.

Gershman, John and Irwin, Alec (2000) Getting a Grip on the Global Economy. In, *Dying for Growth: Global Inequality and the Health of the Poor,* Jim Yong King, Joyce Millen, Alec Irwin and John Gershman, (Eds.) Monroe Maine: Common Courage Press, pp. 11–43.

Gerth, H.H and Mills, C. Wright (1958) *From Max Weber: Essays in Sociology.* New York: Galaxy Books.

Geyer, Georgie Anne (1993) *Guerrilla Prince: The Untold Sotry of Fidel Castro.* Kansas City: Andrews and McMeel.

Gibson-Graham, J.K. (1996) Waiting for the Revolution, or How to Smash Capitalism while Working at Home in Your Spare Time. In, *Marxism in the Postmodern Age: Confronting the New World Order.* Callari, Cullenberg and Biewener, (Eds.) New York: Guilford Press, pp. 188–197.

Gill, AA (1999) Sex and the City. *Sunday Times Magazine.*

Gilpin, Margaret (1991) Cuba: On the Road to a Family Medicine Nation. *Journal of Public Health Policy,* 12(1):83–103.

Gleason, Abbott (1995) *Totalitarianism: The Inner History of the Cold War.* New York: Oxford University Press.

Goff, Fred and Locker, Michael (1969) The Violence of Domination: U.S. Power and the Dominican Republic. In, *Latin American Radicalism,* Irving Louis Horowitz, et al. (Eds.). New York: Random House, pp. 249–291.

Goldscheider, Calvin (1971) *Population, Modernization and Social Structure.* Boston, MA: Little, Brown and Company.

Gott, Richard (2004) *Cuba: A New History.* New Haven, CT: Yale University Press.

Gouré, Leon (1989a) Cuban Military Doctrine and Organization. In, *The Cuban Military Under Castro,* Jaime Suchlicki, (Ed.). Miami, FL: University of Miami North-South Center, pp. 61–91.

Gouré, Leon (1989b) Soviet-Cuban Military Relations. In, *The Cuban Military Under Castro,* Jaime Suchlicki, (Ed.). Miami, FL: University of Miami North-South Center, pp. 165–189.

Graf, William, Hansen, William and Schulz, Brigitte (1993) From The People to One

People: The Social Bases of the East German 'Revolution' and its Pre-emption by the West German State. In, *The Curtain Rises: Rethinking Culture, Ideology and the State in Eastern Europe*. Hermine G. Desoto and David G. Anderson, (Eds.) NJ: Humanities Press, pp. 207–230.

Gruening, Ernest (1931) Cuba under the Machado Regime. *Current History*, 34:214–219.

Guevera Nuñez, Orlando (1997) Una Sola Revolución, Un Mimso Enemigo. *Sierra Maestra*, June 9.

Guggenheim, Harry (1934) *The United States and Cuba*. New York: Macmillon.

Guillemin, Jeanne (1999) *Anthrax: The Investigation of a Deadly Outbreak*. Berkeley, CA: University of California Press.

Guillermoprieto, Alma (1994) *The Heart that Bleeds: Latin America Now*. New York: Alfred A. Knopf.

Gurian, Waldemar (1964) Totalitarianism as Political Religion. In, *Totalitarianism*, Carl J. Friedrich, (Ed.). New York: Grosset and Dunlap, pp. 119–137.

Guiteras, Juan (1962) Papeles de Dr. Juan Guiteras. *Cuaderno de Historia de Salud Publica*, 18. Havana: MINISAP.

Guo, Sujian (1998) The Totalitarian Model Revisited. *Communist and Post-Communist Studies*, 31(3):271–285.

Gustafson, Thane (1997) *Capitalism Russian Style*. Cambridge: Cambridge University Press.

Guttmacher, Sally and Danielson, Ross (1979) Changes in Cuban Health Care: An Argument against Technological Pessimism. *Social Science and Medicine*, 13c:87–96.

Guttmacher, Sally and Garcia, Lourdes (1977) Social Science and Health in Cuba: Ideology, Planning and Health. In, *Topias and Utopias in Health*, Ingram, Stanley and Thomas, Anthony, (Eds.) The Hague: Mouton Publishers, pp. 508–522.

Hahn, Robert and Kleinman, Arthur (1983). Biomedical Practice and Anthropological Theory: Framework and Directions. *Annual Review of Anthropology* 12: 305–333.

Hall, Stuart (1996) Introduction. In, *Modernity: An Introduction to Modern Societies*. Stuart Hall, (Ed.)., London: Blackwell Publishers, pp. 3–18.

Halperin, Maurice (1994) *Return to Havana: The Decline of Cuban Society Under Castro*. Nashville, TN: Vanderbilt University Press.

Hansen, Helena, and Groce, Nora (2003) Human Immunodeficiency Virus and Quarantine in Cuba. *Journal of the American Medical Association*, 290(21):2875–2875.

Hard, William (1928) Charles Evans Hughes, A Pan-American Statesman. *Review of Reviews*, 77:36–48.

Harris, David (2001) *Shooting the Moon*. Boston, MA: Little, Brown and Company.

Harris, Marvin (1999) *Theories of Culture in Postmodern Times*. Walnut Creek, CA: Sage Publications.

Havel, Vaclav (1992) The End of the Modern Era. *New York Times*, March 1.

Hayden, Delores (1978) *Seven American Utopias: The Architecture of Communitarian Socialism*. Cambridge: MIT Press.

Hayek, Friedrich (1944) *The Road to Serfdom*. Chicago, IL: University of Chicago Press.

Haynes, John and Klehr, Harvey (2003) *In Denial: Historians, Communism and Espionage*. San Francisco, CA: Encounter Books.

Hemmes, Michael (1994) Cuba. *Hospitals and Health Networks*, May 5, pp. 52–54.

Henken, Ted (2005) *Entrepreneurship, Informality and the Second Economy: Cuba's Underground Economy in Comparative Perspective*. Paper presented at the 15th annual meeting of the Association for the Study of the Cuban Economy. Miami, Fl.

Hennekens, Charles and Buring, Julie (1987) *Epidemiology in Medicine*. Boston, MA: Little, Brown and Company.

Herrera-Valdéz, R. and Almaguer-López, M. (2005) Strategies for National Health Care Systems and Centers in the Emerging World: Central America and the Caribbean—The Case of Cuba. *Kidney International. Supplement*, 98:s66–68.

Herzog, Arthur (1987) *Vesco*. New York: Doubleday.

Hoch, Steven (1999) Tall Tales: Anthropolmetric Measures of Well-Being in Imperial Russia and the Soviet Union, 1821–1960. *Slavic Review*, spring: 61–70.

Hoernel, Robert (1976) Sugar and Social Change in Oriente, Cuba, 1898–1946. *Journal of Latin American Studies*, 8(2):215–249.

Hollander, Paul (1983) *The Many Faces of Socialism*. New Brunswick, NJ: Transaction Press.

Hollander, Paul (1998[1981] *Political Pilgrims: Western Intellectuals in Search of the Good Society*. New Brunswick, NJ: Transaction Press.

Horowitz, Irving Louis (2003) Military Origin and Evolution of the Cuban Revolution. In, Cuban Communism, 11th edition, Irving Horowitz and Jaime Suchlicki, (Eds.) New Brunswick, NJ: Transaction Press, pp. 388–414.

Horowitz, Irving Louis (1999) *Behemoth: Main Currents in the History and Theory of Political Sociology*. New Brunswick, NJ: Transaction Books.

Horowitz, Irving Louis (1993) *The Decomposition of Sociology*. New York: Oxford University Press.

Horowitz, Irving Louis and Suchlicki, Jaime (2003) Introduction. In, *Cuban Communism*, 11th Edition, Irving Horowitz and Jaime Suchlicki, (Eds.) New Brunswick, NJ: Transaction Press, pp. 3–11.

Huberman, Leo and Sweezy, Paul (1960) *Cuba: Anatomy of a Revolution*. New York: Monthly Review Press.

Human Rights Watch (1999) *Castro's Repressive Machinery*. New York.

Hunt, Richard (1974) *The Political Ideas of Marx and Engeles: Marxism and Totalitarian Democracy, 1818–1850*. Pittsburgh, PA: University of Pittsburgh Press.

Hyatt, John and Hyatt, Pulaski (1898) *Cuba: Its Resources and Opportunities*. New York: Ogilvie.

Infante Marin, Daniel (1997) El Macarthismo de los Anexionistas. *Granma*, February 13.

Infield, Henrik (1955) *Utopia and Experiment: Essays in the Sociology of Cooperation*. Port Washington, DC NY: Kennikat Press.

Ingram, Stanley and Thomas, Anthony (1977) Introduction. In, *Topias and Utopias in Health*.

Ingram, Stanley and Thomas Anthony, (Eds.). The Hague: Mouton Publishers, pp. 1–

20. Instituto Cubano del Libro (1973) *Monopolios Norteamericanos En Cuba*. La Habana: Editorial de Ciencias Sociales.

International Bank for Reconstruction and Development (1950) *Report on Cuba*. Washington, DC.

Isla, Wilfredo Cancio (2005) Crisis en Salud Pública de Cuba. *El Nuevo Herald*. August 15.

James, Daniel (1961) *Cuba: The First Soviet Satellite in the Americas*. New York: Avon Books.

Jenks, Lelend (1929) *Our Cuban Colony*. New York: Vanguard press.

Johsen, Albert, Siegler, Mark, Winslade, William (2002) *Clinical Ethics: A Practical Approach to Ethical Decisions in Clinical Medicine*. New York: McGraw-Hill.

Julien, Claude (1968) *El Imperio Norteamericano*. La Habana: Editorial de Ciencias Sociales.

Kates, Nick (1987) Mental Health Services in Cuba. *Hospital and Community Psychiatry*, 38(7):755–758.

Kellner, Douglas (1996) The End of Orthodox Marxism. In, *Marxism in the Postmodern Age: Confronting the New World Order*. Callari, Cullenberg and Biewener, (Eds.). New York: Guilford Press, pp. 33–41.

Kempe, Frederick (1990) *Divorcing the Dictator: America's Bungled Affair with Noriega*. New York: Putnam's.

Khazanov, Anatoly (1995) *After the U.S.SR: Ethnicity, Nationalism and Politics in the Commonwealth of Independent States*. Madison, WI: University of Wisconsin Press.

Kim, Jim Yong, Shakow, Aaron, Bayona, Jaime et al. (2000) Sickness Amidst Recovery: Public Debt and Private Suffering in Peru. In, *Dying for Growth: Global Inequality and the Health of the Poor*, Jim Yong King, Joyce Millen, Alec Irwin and John Gershman, (Eds.) Monroe, ME: Common Courage Press, pp. 127–154.

Kim, Jim Yong, Millen, Joyce, Irwen, Alec (2000) Introduction. In, *Dying for Growth: Global Inequality and the Health of the Poor*, Jim Yong Kim, Joyce Millen, Alec Irwin and John Gershman, (Eds.) Monroe ME: Common Courage Press, pp. 3–10.

Kirkpatrick, Anthony (2000) U.S. Commits Child Abuse in Cuba. *Miami Herald*. September 5.

Kleinman, Arthur and Kleinman, Joan (1997) Moral Transformations of Health and Suffering in Chinese Society. In *Morality and Health*, Allan Brandt and Paul Rozin, (Eds.) New York: Routledge, pp. 101–118.

Kleinman, Arthur (1986) *Social Origins of Distress and Disease: Depression, Neurasthenia and Pain in Modern China*. New Haven, CT: Yale University Press.

Knaus, William (1981) *Inside Russian Medicine*. Boston, MA: Beacon Press.

Koeves, Tibor (undated) Lucky Luciano Verses the United Nations. Unidentified magazine article located in U.S. Narcotics Bureau files on Lucky Luciano.

Kohak, Erazim (1969) Requiem for Utopia: Socialist Reflections on Czechoslovakia. *Dissent*, January.

Kolakowski, Leszek (1977) Introduction: Need of Utopia, Fear of Utopia. In, *Radicalism in the Contemporary Age, Volume 2: Radical Visions of the Future*, Seweryn Bialer and Sophia Sluzar, (Eds.) Boulder, CO: Westview Press.

Kolakowski, Leszek (1992) Amidst Moving Ruins. *Daedelus*, 121–43–56.

Kourí, Gustavo, Guzmán, Maria Guadalupe, Valdés, Luis et al. (1998) Reemergence of Dengue in Cuba: A 1997 Epidemic in Santiago de Cuba. *Emerging Infectious Diseases,* 4(1):89–92.

Krasner, Stephen (2004) Sharing Sovereignty: New Institutions for Collapsed and Failing States. *International Security*, 29(2):85–120.

Lacey, Robert (1991) *Little Man: Meyer Lansky and the Gangster Life*. Boston, MA: Little, Brown and Company.

Lamar-Schweyer, Alberto (1938) *How President Machado Fell: A Dark Page in North American Diplomacy*. Habana: La Casa Montalvo Cardenas.

Langely, Lester (1989) *The United States and the Caribbean in the Twentieth Century*. Athens, GA: University of Georgia Press.

Lear, Marisela Fleites (2003) Women, Family and the Cuban Revolution. In, *Cuban Communism*, 11th Edition, Iriving Louis Horowitz and Jaime Suchlicki, (Eds.) New Brunswick, NJ: Transaction Press, pp. 276–302.

Ledeneva, Alena (1998) *Russia's Economy of Favors: Blat, Networking and Informal Exchange*. London: Cambridge University Press.

Lenches, Elisabeth Tamedly (1993) The Legacy of Communism: Poisoned Minds and Souls. *International Journal of Social Economics*, 20(5,6,7):14–34.

Leon Cotayo, Nicanor (1997) Unrelenting Crusade against Cuba. *Granma International*. February 5.

Leopold, Evelyn (1999) Modest Heroes get Journalist Award from New York Group. *Cubanet News*, November 23.

Lerner, Michael (1973) *The New Socialist Revolution: An Introduction to its Theory and Strategy*. New York: Dell Books.

LeRoy y Cassá, Jorge (1913) Sanitary Improvement in Cuba as Demonstrated by Statistical Data. *American Journal of Public Health*, 3:255–262.

LeRoy, Jorge (1921) The History of Public Health in Cuba during the Past Fifty Years. *American Journal of Public Health*, 11:1048–1052.

LeRoy y Cassá, Jorge (1922) *Desenvolvimiento de la Sanidad en Cuba durante los Ultimos Años*. Habana: La Moderna Poesía.

Leuchsenring, Emilio Roig (1925) A Disillusioned Cuba. *Living Age*, 324:512–515, March 7.

Levinson, Sandra, Brightman, Carol (1971) *Venceremos Brigade: Young Americans Sharing the Life and work of Revolutionary Cuba*. New York: Simon and Schuster.

Lewis, Ruth (1977) Forward. In, *Four Men: Living the Revolution, An Oral History of Contemporary Cuba*. Chicago, IL: University of Chicago Press, pp. vii-xxxi.

Life Magazine (1958) "Mobsters Move in on Troubled Havana." 44:32–37, March 10.

Lockmiller, David (1938) *Magoon in Cuba: A History of the Second Intervention, 1906–1909*. Chapel Hill: University of North Carolina Press

Lifton, Robert J (1956) Chinese Communist Thought Reform. *Group Processes*, 3:219–312.

Lifton, Robert J. (1961) *Thought Reform and the Psychology of Totalism*. New York: W.W. Norton and Co.

Lifton, Robert Jay (1976) Revolutionary Immortality : Mao Tse-tung and the Chinese Cultural Revolution. New York: WW Norton and Company.

Lindsey, Forbes (1911) *Cuba and her People of Today.* Boston: L.L. Page and Co.

Lockmiller, David (1938) *Magoon in Cuba: A History of the Second Intervention, 1906–1909.* Chapel Hill, NC: University of North Carolina Press.

Lopez de Valle (1924) *Los Adelantes Sanitarios de la República de Cuba.* La Havana: Imprenta y Papelaria "La Propagandista."

Lopez del Valle (1927) *Legislación y Organización Sanitaria y de Beneficia de la republica de Cuba.* Habana: Libreria a Nueva Pi y Morgall.

López Leiva, Fransisco (1930) *El Bandolerismo en Cuba.* La Habana: Imprenta El Siglo XX.

Lopez Silvero, J.E. (1926) A Statistical Survey of the Sanitary Condition of Cuba. *American Journal of Public Health,* 16:1214–1217.

Lopez Silvero, J.E. (1930) Cuban Sanitary and Hospital Activities. *Southern Medical Journal,* 23(1):37–40.

Louw, Stephen (1997) Unity and Development: Social Homogeneity, the Totalitarian Imaginary and the Classical Marxist Tradition. *Philosophy of the Social Sciences,* 27(2):180–205.

Lowinger, Rosa and Fox, Ofelia (2005) *Tropicana Nights: The Life and Times of the Legendary Cuban Nightclub.* Orlando, FL: Harcourt.

Löwy, Michael (1992) *Marxism in Latin America from 1909 to the Present.* N J: Humanities Press.

Llovio-Menéndez, José (1988) *Insider: My Hidden Life as a Revolutionary In Cuba.* Toronto: Bantam Books.

Luce, Phillip Abbot (1971) *The New Left Today.* Washington, DC: Capitol Hill Press.

Lumen, Enrique (1935) *La Revolucion Cubana.* Mexico City: Ediciones Botas.

Lynch, Grayston (1998) *Decision for Disaster: Betrayal at the Bay of Pigs.* Washington, DC: Brasseys.

Lyons, Paul (1975) The New Left and the Cuban Revolution. In, *The New Cuba: Paradoxes and Potentials,* Radosh, Ronald, (Ed.). New York: William Morrow, pp. 211–246.

Magoon, Charles (1909) Final Report to President following the second U.S. Military Occupation of Cuba. Havana April 16th.

Malia, Martin (1994) *The Soviet Tragedy: A History of Socialism in Russia, 1917–1991.* New York: The Free Press.

Manuel, Frank (1992) A Requiem for Karl Marx. *Daedelus,* 121:1–21.

Marrerroa, Antonio, Caminerob, José, Rodriguez, Rodolfo and Billob, Nils (2000) Toward Elimination of Tuberculosis in a Low Income Country: The Experience of Cuba. *Thorax,* 55:39–45.

Marshall, Jeffery (1998) The Political Viability of Free Market Experimentation in Cuba: Evidence from Los Mercados Agropecuarios. *World Development,* 26(2):277–288.

Martino, John (1963) *I Was Castro's Prisoner.* New York: Devin Adair Company.

Massetti, Jorge (1993) *In the Pirate's Den: My Life as a Secret Agent for Castro.* San Francisco, CA: Encounter Books.

Mathews, Franklin (1899) *The New Born Cuba.*

Matthews, Herbert (1952) Republic with no Citizens. *New York Times Magazine,* May 18, p. 12

Matthews, Herbert (1961) *The Cuban Story*. New York: George Braziller.

McKeown, Thomas (1976) *The Role of Medicine: Dream, Mirage or Nemesis?* London:

Mead, Margaret (1951) *Soviet Attitudes Toward Authority: An Interdisciplinary Apprach to Problem of Soviet Character*. New York: Schocken Books.

Mechanic, David (1976) *The Growth of Bureaucratic Medicine: An Inquiry into the Dynamics of Patient Behavior and the Organization of Medical Care*. New York: Wiley and Sons.

Mencia, Manuel (1936) *La Sanidad y La Beneficia en Cuba: Reformas Indispensables*. La Habana: Molines y Compania.

Mendoza, Dessy Rivero and Fuentes, Ileana (2001) *¡Dengue!* Washington, DC: Center for a Free Cuba.

Miliband, Ralph (1996) Reclaiming the Alternative. In, *Marxism in the Postmodern Age: Confronting the New World Order*. Callari, Cullenberg and Biewener, (Eds.) New York: Guilford Press, pp. 218–224.

Millar, James (1987) *Politics, Work and Daily life in the U.S.S.R.* Cambridge: Cambridge University Press.

Miller, Warren (1961) *Ninety Miles from Home: The Truth From Inside Castro's Cuba*. New York: Faucett Books.

Mills, C. Wright (1961) *Listen Yankee: The Revolution in Cuba*. New York: Ballantine Books.

MINISAP (1960) *Subdesarrollo Economico, principal enemigo de la Salud—Como Lo Combate La Revolucion Cubana*. Habana.

MINISAP (1961) *Desarrollo Economico y Salud en Cuba Revolucionario*. Habana.

MINISAP (1963) *Plan de Trabajo para Los Responsables de Salud de los CDR*. Habana.

MINISAP (1968) *La Ofensiva Revolucionaria en Salud Publica*. Habana.

MINISAP (1969) *Diez Años de Revolución en Salud Publica*. Habana: Editorial de Ciencias Sociales.

MINISAP (1974) *Cuba—Organizacion de los Servicios y Nivel de Salud*. Habana.

MINISAP (1979) *Coleccion del Estudiante de Medicina: Introduccion a la Especialidad*. La Habana.

MINISAP (1986) *Sociedad y Salud*. La Habana.

MINISAP (1997) Fact Sheet on Health Trends in Oriente Province since 1959. Prepared for the Third Annual International Symposium on Health Economics.

Ministerio de Salubridad y Asistencia Social (1953) *Un Año de labor Sanitaria y Hospitaliria*. Habana.

Mintz, Sidney (1966 [1964]) The Industrialization of Sugar Production and its Relationship to Social and Economic Change. In, Smith, Robert F. (Ed.), *Background to Revolution: the Development of Modern Cuba*. New York: Alfred Knopf, pp. 176–186.

Molina, Gabriel (1997) From Colony to Neocolony. *Granma Internacional*, June 15, pp. 8–10.

Mommsen, Wolfgang (1977) Max Weber as a Critic of Marxism. *Canadian Journal of Sociology*, 2(4):373–398.

Mommsen, Wolfgang (1980) *Theories of Imperialism*. Chicago, IL: University of Chicago Press.

Montaner, Carlos Alberto (1981) *Secret Report on the Cuban Revolution*. New Brunswick, NJ: Transaction Press.

Montaner, Carlos Alberto (1985) *Cuba, Castro and the Caribbean*. New Brunswick, NJ: Transaction Press.

Montaner, Carlos Alberto (2005) Slaves in White Coats. *Miami Herald*, September 13.

Moore, Carlos (1986) Congo or Caribalí? Race Relations in Socialist Cuba. *Caribbean Review*, 15(2):12–15.

Morin, Emilio Ichikawa (2003) The Moral Basis of Cuban Society. In, *Cuban Communism*, 11th Edition, Irving Louis Horowitz and Jaime Suchlicki, (Eds.) New Brunswick: Transaction Press, pp. 329–340.

Mormino, Gary and Pozzetta, George (1998 [1990]) *The Immigrant World of Ybor City: Italians and their Latin Neighbors in Tampa, 1885–1985*. Gainesville, FL: University of Florida Press.

Morris, James A. (1989) Introduction. In, *The Cuban Military Under Castro*, Jaime Suchlicki, (Ed.). Miami, FL: University of Miami North-South Center Publications, pp. xvi-xviii.

Moses, Catherine (2000) *Real Life in Castro's Cuba*. Washington, DC: Scholarly Resources.

Muller, H.J. (1964) Science under Soviet Totalitarianism. In, *Totalitarianism*, Carl J. Friedrich, ((Ed.).) New York: Grosset and Dunlap, pp. 233–244.

National Institute for Savings and Gambling (1959) *Revolutionary Reform of Gambling*. Havana.

Navarro, Vincente (1972) Health, Health Services and Health Planning in Cuba. *International Journal of Health Services*, 3(2):397–432.

Navarro, Vincente (1976) *Medicine Under Capitalism*. New York: Prodist.

Navarro, Vincente (1978). *Class Struggle, The State and Medicine*. New York, Prodist.

Navarro, Vincente (1986) *Crisis, Health and Medicine*. New York: Tavistock.

Navarro, Vincente (1989) Radicalism, Marxism and Medicine. *Medical Anthropology*, 11:195–219.

Nayeri, Kamran (1995) The Cuban Health Care System and Factors Currently Undermining It. *Journal of Community Health*, 20(4):321–334.

Newman, Lucia (1997) Few Independent Journalists Challenge Cuba's Restrictions. *CNN Interactive*, March 18.

Norton, Albert (1900) *Norton's complete hand-book of Havana and Cuba*. Chicago, IL: Rand McNally and Co.

Norton, Henry Kittredge (1926) Self-Determination in the West-Indies. *World's Work*, 51:76–84; 210–218; 321–328.

Oglesby, Carl (1969) Introduction: The Idea of the New Left. In, *The New Left Reader*, Carl Oglesby, (Ed.). New York: Grove Press, pp. 1–20.

Onoge, Omafume (1977) Capitalism and Public Health: A Neglected Theme in the Medical Anthropology of Africa. In, *Topias and Utopias in Health*, Ingram, Stanely and Thomas, Anthony, (Eds.) The Hague: Mouton Publishers, pp. 220–232.

Oppenheimer, Andres (1993) *Castro's Final Hour*. New York: Touchstone Books.

Ortega, Francisco (1940) *Informe al Hon. Señor Secretario de Sanidad y Beneficia acerca de los Trabajos Realizados al frente de la Jefatura Local de Santiago de Cuba*. Habana.

Ortiz, Fernando (1924) *La Decadencia Cubana*. Habana: Imprenta La Universal.

Padillla, Heberto (1984) *Heroes are Grazing in My Garden*. New York: Farrar, Straus and Giroux.

Padula, Alfred (1993) Cuban Socialism: Thirty Years of Controversy. In, *Conflict and Change in Cuba*, Enrique Baloyra and James Morris, (Eds.) Albuquerque: University of New Mexico Press, pp. 15–37.

Paterson, Thomas (1994) *Contesting Castro: The United States and the Cuban Revolution*. New York: Oxford University Press.

Paz, Octavio (1990) *The Other Voice: Essays on Modern Poetry*. San Diego, CA: Harcourt Brace Jovanovich.

Pelto, B. (1988). A Note on Critical Medical Anthropology. *Medical Anthropology Quarterly* 2:

Perez, Louis (1978) *Intervention, Revolution and Politics in Cuba, 1913–1921*. Pittsburgh, PA: University of Pittsburgh Press.

Perez, Louis (1983) *Cuba Between Empires 1878–1902*. Pittsburgh, PA: University of Pittsburgh Press.

Perez, Louis (1986) *Cuba Under the Platt Amendment, 1902–1934*. Pittsburgh, PA: University of Pittsburgh Press.

Perez, Louis (1988) *Cuba: Between Reform and Revolution*. New York: Oxford University Press.

Perez Louis (1995) *Essays on Cuban History*. Gainesville, FL: University of Florida Press.

Pérez-López, Jorge (2002) The Cuban Economy in an Unending Special Period.

Perez-Lopez, Jorge (1995) *Cuba's Second Economy*. New Brunswick, NJ: Transaction Press.

Perez-Lopez, Jorge (1997) Cuba's Second Economy and the Market Transition. In, *Toward a New Cuba: Legacies of a Revolution*, Centeno, Miguel and Font, Mauricio, (Eds.), Boulder, CO: Lynn Rienner, pp. 171–186.

Perez-Stable, Marifeli (1993) *The Cuban Revolution: Origins, Course and Legacy*. New York: Oxford University Press.

Peters, Phillip, and Scarpaci, Joseph (1998) *Cuba's New Entrepreneurs: Fivce Years of Small-Scale Capitalism*. Arlington, VA: Alex De Tocqueville Institiue.

Phillips, Ruby Hart (1935) *Cuban Sideshow*. Havana: Cuba Press.

Phillips, Ruby Hart (1949) Cuba Plans to End Rebellious Gangs. *New York Times*. October 9

Phillips, Ruby Hart (1959) *Cuba: Island of Paradox*. New York: McDowell Obolensky.

Pierre, Fidel (1896) *Cuba*. New York: Cuban Delegation to the United States.

Pilisuk, Marc (1984) The Dominican Counterexample to Cuba: The American Path to Development. *International Journal of Health Services*, 14(2):217–235.

Pino-Santos, Oscar (1964) *Historia de Cuba: Aspectos Fundamentales*. La Habana: Editoria Universitaria.

Portal, Manuel (1998) 'Asere', en Cuba no te dejan vivir. *El Nuevo Herald*, November 22.

Porter, Robert. *Industrial Cuba* (1899) New York: Putnams.

Pratt, Julius (1950) *America's Colonial Experiments*. New York: Prentice-Hall.

Radosh, Ronald (2001) *Commies: A Journey Through the Old, Left, the New Left and the Leftover Left*. San Francisco, CA: Encounter Books.

Ragano, Frank and Raab, Selwyn (1994) *Mob Lawyer*. New York: Scribners.

Randall, Margaret (1981) *Women in Cuba: Twenty Years Later*. New York: Smyrna Press.

Rea, George Bronson (1897) *Facts and Fakes about Cuba*. New York: George Munro.

Recio, Alberto (1945) *Enfermedades Infecto-Contagiosas que Amenazan a Cuba. Anales de la Academía de Ciencias Medicas, Fisicas y Naturales de la Habana*. Habana.

Remington, Thomas (1988) *The Truth of Authority: Ideology and Communication in the Soviet Union*. Pittsburgh, PA: University of Pittsburgh Press.

Rieff, David (1994) *The Exiles: Cuba in the Heart of Miami*. New York: Simon and Schuster.

Ries, Nancy (1997) *Russian Talk*. Ithaca, NY: Cornell University Press.

Rigol, Orlando Ricardo, Perez, Francicso Carballás, Perea, Jesús Sacasas y Fernández, José Miabal (1994) *Medicina General Integral—Tomo Uno*. La Habana: Editorial Pueblo y Educación.

Ring, Harry (1961) *How Cuba Uprooted Race Discimination*. New York: Pioneer Publishers.

Ritter, Archibald (2005) *Survival Strategies and Economic Illegalities in Cuba, 2005: Character, Causes, Consequences and Cures*. Paper presented at the 15th annual meeting of the Association for the Study of the Cuban Economy. Miami, FL, July 2995.

Robert, W. Adolphe (1953) *Havana: Portrait of a City*. New York: Coward-McLann.

Roca, Sergio (1993) The Commandante in his Economic Labryinth. In, *Conflict and Change in Cuba*, Baloyra, Enrique and Morris, James, (Eds.) Albuquerque: University of New Mexico Press, pp. 86–109.

Rodruiguez Alvarez, Angel (1997) No Podrán Demarmar a Nuestro Pueblo, Dividirlo y Esclavisarlo. *Granma*, Februrary 28.

Rodriguez, Leonel Cordova and Martinez, Noris Pena (2000) Testimony before U.S. Senate Foreign Relations Committee, United States Senate. September 20, 2000.

Rofes, Sunset Nogueras (2000) Lies in Death Certificates Manipulate Statistics. *CubaNet News*, June 19.

Rogers, Richard and Hackenberg, Robert (1987) Extending Epidemiological Transition Theory: A New Stage. *Social Science and Medicine*, 34(3–4):234–243.

Roig, Emilio de Leuschenring (1925) A Disillusioned Cuba. *Living Age*, 324:512–515, March 7.

Rojas, Marta (1986) *El Medico de la Familia en La Sierra Maestra*. La Habana: Editorial Ciencias Medicas.

Román, Gustavo (1994) Epidemic Neuropathy in Cuba. *Neurology*, 44:1784–1786.

Rose-Ackerman, Susan (1978) *Corruption: A Study in Political Economy*. New York: Academic Press.

Rosendahl, Mona (1997) *Inside the Revolution: Everyday Life in Socialist Cuba.* Ithaca, NY: Cornell University Press.

Rosenberg, Tina (1996) *The Haunted Land: Facing Europe's Ghosts After Communism.* New York: Vintage Books.

Rosengarten, Frank (1996) Was the Soviet Union Socialist? In, *Marxism in the Postmodern Age: Confronting the New World Order.* Callari, Cullenberg and Biewener, (Eds.) New York: Guilford Press, pp. 333–341.

Rovner, Eduardo Saenz (2004) *Contrabando, Juego y Narcotrafico en Cuba entre los Años 20 y Comienzos de la Revolucion.* Paper presented at Cátedra UNESCO, Transformaciones económicas y sociales relacionadas con el problema internacional de las drogas, Instituto de Investigaciones sociales de la Unam, Mexico, March 17.

Safa, Helen (1995) *The Myth of the Male Breadwinner.* Boulder, CO: Westview Press.

Sakharov, Vladimir (1980) *High Treason.* New York: Ballantine Books.

Salvadori, Massimo (1968) Introduction. In, *Modern Socialism.* Salvadori, ed, pp. 1–38.

Santana, Sarah (1988) Some Thoughts on Vital Statistics and Health Status in Cuba. In, *Cuban Political Economy: Controversies in Cubanology*, Andrew Zimbalist, (Ed.). Boulder. CO: Westview Press, pp. 107–118.

Sartre, Jean-Paul (1961) *Sartre on Cuba.* New York: Ballantine Books.

Scheper-Hughes, Nancy (1990) Three Propositions for a Critically Applied Medical Anthropology. *Social Science and Medicine*, 30(2):189–197.

Scheper-Hughes, Nancy (1993) AIDS, Public Health and Human Rights in Cuba. *The Lancet*, 342:965–968.

Schneider, M.C., Castillo-Salgado, C., Loyola-Elizondo, E.et al. (2002) Trends in Infant Mortality in the Americas, 1955–1995. *Journal of Epidemiology and Community Health*, 56:538–541.

Schutz, Barry (1995) The Heritage of Revolution and the Struggle for Governmental Legitimacy in Mozambique. In, Zartman, William, (Ed.). *Collaped) States: The Disintegration and Restoration of Legitimate Authority.* Boulder: Lynne Reinner, pp. 109–124.

Schiffres, Manuel (1998) A Capitalist in Cuba. *Kiplinger's Personal Finance Magazine*, 52(3):150–154.

Schwartz, Rosalie (1989) *Lawless Liberators: Political Banditry and Cuban Independence.* Durham, NC: Duke University Press.

Scott, James (1972) *Comparative Political Corruption.* Englewood Cliffs, NJ: Prentice-Hall.

Secretaria de Sanidad y Beneficia (1931) *Cinco Años de Labor Sanitaria y de Beneficencia Publica.* La Habana: Emprenta y Libreria La Propaganda.

Serviet, Pedro (1993) Solutions to the Black Problem. In *AfroCuba: An Anthropology of Cuban Writing on Race, Politics and Culture*, Perez Sarduy, Pedro and Stubbs, Jean, (Eds.), pp. 77–90.

Sidel, Victor and Sidel, Ruth (1977) The Health Care Delivery System of the People's Republic of China. In, *Health by the People*, Kenneth Newell, (Ed.). Geneva: World Health Organization, pp. 1–13.

Silvero, Jose (1926) A Statistical Survey of the Sanitary Condition in Cuba. *American Journal of Public Health*, 16:1214–1217.

Simons, Geoff (1996) *Cuba: From Conquistador to Castro.* New York: St. Martin's Press.

Singer, Merrill (1990) Reinventing Medical Anthropology: Toward a Critical Realignment. *Social Science and Medicine,* 30(2):v-viii.

Singer, Merrill and Baer Hans (1995) *Critical Medical Anthropology.* Amityville: Baywood.

Singer, Merrill and Baer, Hans (1989) Toward an Understanding of Capitalist and Socialist Health. *Medical Anthropology,* 11:97–102.

Singer, Merrill, Baer, Hans and Lazarus, Ellen (Eds.) (1990) Critical Medical Anthropology: Theory and Method. *Social Science and Medicine,* 30:2.

Singer, Merrill, Valentín, Freddie, Baer, Hans and Jia Zhongke (1992) Why Does Juan Garcia have a Drinking Problem? The Perspective of Critical Medical Anthropology. *Medical Anthropology,* 13:77–108.

Simonelli, Jeanne (1987) Defective Modernization and Health in Mexico. *Social Science and Medicine,* 24(1):23–36.

Sirc, Ljubo (1994) *Why the Communist Economies Failed.* London: Center for Research into Communist Economics.

Smith, Kirby and Llorens, Hugo (1998) Renaissance and Decay: A Comparison of Socioeconomic Indicators in Pre-Castro and Current-Day Cuba. Paper presented at the Eigth Annual Meeting of the Association for the Study of the Cuban Economy, Coral Gables, FL.

Smith, Theresa and Oleszczuk, Thomas (1996) *No Asylum: State Psychiatric Repression in the Former U.S.S.R.* London: Macmillon.

Smith, Wayne (1996) Cuba's Long Reform. *Foreign Affairs,* 75(2):99–112.

Smith, Lois and Padula, Afred (1996) *Sex and Revolution: Women in Socialist Cuba.* New York: Oxford University Press.

Solzhenitsyn, Alexander (1973) *The Gulag Archipelago.* New York: Harper and Row.

Solzhenitsyn, Alexander (1976) *Warning to the West.* New York: Farrar, Straus and Giroux.

Sontag, Susan (1969) Some Thoughts on the Right Way (for us) to Love the Cuban Revolution. *Ramparts,* April:6–19.

Spiegel, J.M. and Yassi, A. (2004) Lessons from the Margins of Globalization: Appreciating the Cuban Health Paradox. *Journal of Public Health Policy,* 25(1):85–110.

Spinden, Herbert (1920) Shall the United States Intervene in Cuba? *World's Work,* 41:465–483.

Stephen, Nancy (1977) *Interactions between Socio-Economic and Political factors and Medical Science.* Yale University.

Stokes, William. (1966) National and Local Violence in Cuban Politics. In Smith, Robert F. (Ed.)., *Background to Revolution: the Development of Modern Cuba.* New York: Alfred Knopf, pp. 142–148.

Suchlicki, Jaime (2000) Castro's Cuba: Continuity Instead of Change. In *Cuba: The Contours of Change,* Kaufman Purcell, Susan and Rothkopf, David, (Eds.) Boulder: Lynne Rienner, pp. 57–80.

Suchlicki, Jaime (1969) *University Students and Revolution in Cuba, 1920–1968.* Coral Gables, FL: University of Miami Press.

Suchlicki, Jaime (1997) *Cuba: From Columbus to Castro and Beyond.* Washington, DC: Brassey's.

Suchlicki, Jaime (1993) Myths and Realities in U.S.-Cuban Relations. *Journal of Interamerican Studies and World Affairs,* 35(2):103–113.

Spiegel, Jerry and Yassi, Annalee (2004) Lessons from the Margins of Globalization: Appreciating the Cuban Health Paradox. *Journal of Public Health Policy,* 25(1):85–110.

Suárez, Andrés (1989) Civil-Military Relations in Cuba. In, *The Cuban Military Under Castro,* Jaime Suchlicki, (Ed.). Miami, FL: University of Miami North-South Center, pp. 129–160.

Swanson, Karen, Swanson, Janice, Gill, Ayesha, and Walter, Chris (1995) Primary Care in Cuba: A Public Health Approach. *Health Care for Women International,* 16:299–308.

Sweezy, Paul (1949) *Socialism.* New York: McGraw-Hill.

Szaz, Ivan (1987) Health Care in Cuba: "I Left with a Strong Sense of Respect." *CMAJ,* 137:441–443.

Talmon, JL (1960) *Political Messianism: The Romantic Phase.* London: Secker and Warburg.

Talmon, J.L. (1967) *Romanticism and Revolt: Europe 1815–1848.* New York: WW Norton and Company.

Tamayo, Juan (2002) Cuba's Last Gamble? *Miami Herald.* April 8.

Tanzi, Vito (1995) Corruption: Arm's Length Relationships and Markets. In, *The Economics of Organized Crime,* Gianluca Fiorentini and Sam Peltzman, (Eds.) Cambridge: Cambridge University Press, pp. 161–180.

Taussig, Michael (1974) Nutrition, Development, and Foreign Aid: A Case Study of U.S. Directed Health Care in a Colombian Plantation Zone. *Imperialism, Health and Medicine,* Navarro, Vincente, (Ed.). Farmindale, NY: Baywood, pp. 127–147.

Taussig, Michael (1980) Reification and the Consciousness of the Patient. *Social Science and Medicine,* 14b:3–13.

Terry, Philip T. (1929) *Terry's Guide to Cuba.* Boston: Houghton Mifflin Co.

Therborn, Goran (1992) The Life and Times of Socialism. *New Left Review,* 194:17–32.

Thomas, Anthony (1977) Health Care in Ukambani Kenya: A Socialist Critique. In, *Topias and Utopias in Health,* Ingram, Stanely and Thomas, Anthony, (Eds.) The Hague: Mouton Publishers, pp. 267–281.

Thomas, Hugh (1998 [1972]) *Cuba: The Pursuit of Freedom.* New York: Harper and Row.

Thomas, Hugh (2001) Cuba: The United States and Batista, 1952–1958. In, *Cuban Communism,* 11th Edition, Irving Louis Horowitz, (Ed.). New Brunswick, NJ: Transaction Press, pp. 12–20.

Timerman, Jacobo (1990) *Cuba: A Journey.* New York: Alfred Knopf.

Trouillot, Michel-Rolph (1990) *State Against Nation: The Origins and Legacy of Duvaliarism.* New York: Monthly Review Press.

Tulchinsky, Theodore and Varavikova, Elena (1996) Addressing the Epidemiologic Transition in the Former Soviet Union: Strategies for Health System and Public Health Reform in Russia. *American Journal of public Health,* 86(3):313–320.

Turner, Curtis (1932) *Cuba Under the Platt Amendment*. Masters thesis, Emory College.

United States Department of Justice (1998) U.S. Dismantles Largest Global Alien Suggling Cartel Encountered to Date. Washington, DC.

United States Department of State, Bureau of Public Affairs (1985) *Case Study of Cuban Hypocrisy: The 1981 Dengue Epidemic in Cuba*. Washington, DC: Special Report #133.

United States Information Agency (1985) *In a Place Without a Soul: The Testimony of Former Cuban Political Prisoners*. Washington, DC.

United States Senate (1960) *Communist Threat to the United States Through the Caribbean*. Hearings Before the Subcommittee to Investigate the Administration of the Internal Security act and Other Internal Security Laws of the Committee on the Judiciary. 86th Congress. Second Session. Part 9. August 27, 30.

Valdés, Julio (1997) Economic Changes in Cuba: Problems and Challenges. In, *Toward a New Cuba: Legacies of a Revolution*, Centeno, Miguel and Font, Mauricio, (Eds.), Boulder, CO: Lynn Rienner, pp. 187–200.

Valladares, Armando (1986) *Against All Hope*. New York: Ballantine Books.

Van Voren (1989) *Soviet Psychiatric Abuse in the Gorbachev Era*. Amsterdam: International Association on the Political Use of Psychiatry.

Verdery, Katherine (1996) *What Was Socialism and What Comes Next?* Princeton, NJ: Princeton University Press.

Verdery, Katherine (1999) Introduction. In, *Uncertain Transitions: Ethnographies of Change in the Postsocialist World*. Burawoy and Verdery, (Eds.) Boulder, CO: Rowman and Littlefield, pp. 1–19.

Waitzkin, Howard (1983) *The Second Sickness: Contradictions of Capitalist Health Care*. New York: The Free Press.

Waitzkin, Howard and Britt, Theron (1989) Changing the Structure of Medical Discourse: Implications of Cross-National Comparisons. *Journal of Health and Social Behavior*, 30:436–449.

Waitzkin, Howard, Wald, K., Kee, R., et al. (1997) Primary Care in Cuba: Low and High-Technology Developments Pertinent to Family Medicine. *Journal of Family Practice*, 45(3):250–258.

Wald, Karen (1978) *Children of Che: Childcare and Education in Cuba*. Palo Alto, CA: Ramparts Press.

Wald, Karin (1989) Cuban Women Face the Future. *The Black Scholar*, 20(5–6):14–16.

Walker, Phyllis Greene (1989) Cuban Military Service System: Organization, Obligations and Pressures. In, *The Cuban Military Under Castro*, Jaime Suchlicki, (Ed.). Miami, FL: University of Miami North-South Center, pp. 99–126.

Walker, Phyllis Greene (1993) Political-Military Relations since 1959. In, *Conflict and Change in Cuba*, Enrique A. Baloyra and James Morris, (Eds.) Albuquerque: University of New Mexico Press, pp. 110–136.

Waller, J. Michael and Yasmann, Victor (1995) Russia's Great Criminal Revolution: The Role of the Security Services. *Journal of Contemporary Criminal Justice*, 11(4):

Warman, Andrea (2001) Living the Revolution: Cuban Health Workers. *Journal of Clinical Nursing*, 10:311–319.

Waters, Mary-Alice (1989) Cuba: A Historic Moment. *The Black Scholar*, 20(5–6):2–4.

Whiteford, Linda (2000) Local Identity, Globalization and Health in Cuba and the Dominican Republic. In, *Global Health Policy, Local Realities: The Fallacy of the Level Playing Field.* Linda Whiteford and Lenore Manderson, (Eds.) Boulder, CO: Lynn Reimer Press, pp. 57–78.

Whiteford, Linda and Martinez, Dinorah (2001) *The Cuban Health Care System: The Challenge of Success.* Paper presented at the Cuban Research Institute, Miami, FL.

Wiarda, Howard (1968) *Dictatorship and Development: The Methods of Social Control in Trujillo's Dominican Republic.* Gainesville, FL: Center for Latin American Studies.

Wolf, Eric and Hansen, Edward (1966) Caudillo Politics, A Structural Analysis. *Comparative Studies in Society and History,* 9:168–179.

Woon, Basil Dillon (1929) *When It's Cocktail Time in Cuba.* New York: H. Liveright.

Wraith, Ronald and Simkins, Edgar (1963) *Corruption in Developing Countries.* New York: Norton and Co.

Wright, Irene (1910) *Cuba.* New York: MacMillan.

Wright, Thomas (2001) *Latin American in the Era of the Cuban Revolution.* Westport, CT: Praeger.

Wrong, Dennis (1962) The American Left and Cuba. *Commentary,* February pp. 93–103.

Yglesias, Jose (1969) *In the Fist of the Revolution: Life in a Cuban Country Town.* New York: Random House.

Zartman, William (1995) Introduction. In, Zartman, William, (Ed.) *Collapsed States: The Disintegration and Restoration of Legitimate Authority.* Boulder, CO: Lynne Reinner, pp. 1–14.

Zimbalist, Andrew (2000) Whiter the Cuban Economy? In, *Cuba: The Contours of Change,* Susan Purcell and David Rothkopf, (Eds.) Boulder, CO: Lynn Rienner Press, pp. 13–30.

Zimbalist, Andrew and Eckstein, Susan (1987) Patterns of Cuban Development: The First Twenty-Five Years." In, *Cuba's Socialist Economy Toward the 1990s,* Zimbalist, Andrew, (Ed.). Boulder, CO: Lynne Rienner.

Index

Printed in the United States
by Baker & Taylor Publisher Services